Aromatherapy
A NATURAL CHOICE

LIZA NAGY

HODDER

Essential oils are very powerful therapeutic substances and must be treated with respect. The purpose of this book is to help you make informed decisions in regard to your health. It is not offered as a medical reference book. Neither the author nor the publisher can be held responsible should any adverse reactions occur as a result of the use of any of the recipes, formulas, recommendations or instructions contained herein.

Self diagnosis or self treatment should not be attempted for serious or long term illnesses without first seeking the opinion of a professionally qualified aromatherapist or medical practitioner. Do not substitute aromatherapy for medically prescribed treatments without first seeking professional advice.

Experience has shown that each person reacts uniquely and individually to any health maintenance program, be it aromatherapy or otherwise. Therefore no guarantes of any kind are made or implied as to the effectiveness of any of the preparations or procedures mentioned herein.

General editor: Pamela Allardice
Editors: Elizabeth Neate, Tom Gilliatt
Designer: Liz Seymour
Illustrator: Chris Wilson

A Hodder & Stoughton Book

First published in Australia and New Zealand in 1995
by Hodder Headline Australia Pty Limited
(A member of the Hodder Headline Group)
10–16 South Street, Rydalmere NSW 2116

Originally titled The Natural Choice Guide to Aromatherapy

This edition published in 1998

Copyright © 1995 by Liza Nagy

This book is copyright. Apart from any fair dealing for the purposes of private study, research, criticism or review as permitted under the Copyright Act 1968, no part may be stored or reproduced by any process without prior written permission. Enquiries should be made to the publisher.

National Library of Australia Cataloguing-in-Publication data
Nagy, Liza
  Aromatherapy a natural choice

  New ed.
  ISBN 0 7336 1014 5.

  1. Aromatherapy. 2. Essences and essential oils —
  Therapeutic use. I. Title.

615.321

Typeset in 12/14 Bembo by Midland Typesetters, Maryborough
Printed and bound in Australia by Griffin Press, Adelaide

CONTENTS

Foreword V
Measuring Ingredients VII

CHAPTER 1 ➤
ESSENTIAL OILS *1*

CHAPTER 2 ➤
SOME FACTS ABOUT AROMATHERAPY *23*

CHAPTER 3 ➤
AROMATHERAPY FOR BABIES AND YOUNG CHILDREN *32*

CHAPTER 4 ➤
AROMATHERAPY FOR TEENAGERS *52*

CHAPTER 5 ➤
AROMATHERAPY FOR WOMEN *72*

CHAPTER 6 ➤
AROMATHERAPY FOR MEN *92*

CHAPTER 7 ➤
AROMATHERAPY AND SPORT *111*

CHAPTER 8 ➤
MAKE YOUR OWN AROMATHERAPY BEAUTY PRODUCTS *124*

CHAPTER 9 ➤
A–Z GUIDE TO ESSENTIAL OILS *141*

Glossary 177
Further reading 179
Index 181

ACKNOWLEDGMENTS

'Sunshine', *thanks for your invaluable feedback. Thanks also to family, friends, individuals and organisations who assisted with support, constructive opinions and information. And, a self-pat, for doing it!*

FOREWORD

Standing in a health food store one day, I noticed two women approach an aromatherapy range comprising around thirty beautifully packaged essential oils. One picked up a bottle, smelt it with delight, then asked, 'What do you do with them? Drop them in your mouth?'! This lack of knowledge could have been potentially harmful. Essential oils when used with care (mainly externally) can have wide-ranging benefits:

Emotionally, they can uplift and motivate, or calm and relieve tension to help you feel good again.

Physically, they can assist in the healing of many ailments (see summary charts in Chapter 9).

They should never be used internally without the advice of a qualified aromatherapist.

This book was born from the many questions budding aromatherapy enthusiasts have asked me during my numerous Beginners workshops. It presumes you know nothing about the subject. It teaches you how to distinguish between 'pure' essential oils and synthetic ones; it tells you how essential oils work and why, and how to shop for and store them; it gives you aromatherapy 'recipes' for situations and ailments that are common to each stage of life; it shows you basic massage techniques, and how to make your own aromatherapy beauty products at home; and it tells you about the emotional and physical benefits of around thirty essential oils so that you can enjoy the challenge of making your own blends.

Before I studied aromatherapy I looked at a few aromatherapy books and was terribly confused. They seemed to recommend different essential oils for the same ailments and have different blending recipes. After studying the subject I can see why. So, to help you avoid confusion, let me explain.

There are several essential oils that can assist in healing the one ailment. For example, bergamot, cedarwood, chamomile, geranium, lavender, marjoram, neroli, orange, patchouli, petitgrain and sandalwood are all essential oils used to treat mild depression. In most 'recipes' you will seldom see more than three of these in an aromatherapy blend. The essential oil selection can obviously vary between books.

The number of drops in a blend may also vary slightly from book to book. An aromatherapist's personal experience or preference may also influence the finished product. In this book I have deliberately used different techniques and quantities (utilising the standard formula for blending) to give you various examples. The recipes are only for guidance; you could choose different base oils or essential oils in the blends.

While we're on blending, the 'notes' of essential oils (see Chapter 9) may also vary in some cases. For example, some say lavender is a 'top' note while others say it is a 'middle' note. By this you can assume that lavender is between a top and a middle note. Use Chapter 9 as a reference, and please read the 'Safety' section in the description of each essential oil before making a blend, until you become familiar with the subject.

As a naturopath who is qualified in medical herbalism, I was fascinated by the difference between the therapeutic action of the whole plant versus the essential oil component. Sometimes it is very similar. But, if you have knowledge of herbs, do not assume that the essential oil will have the same healing qualities as the plant.

With more knowledge and experience, I found that the aromatherapy books I had originally looked at made perfect sense. If you have any questions, ask your local aromatherapist for advice. If you have a specific ailment or want to discover the benefits of a luxurious aromatherapy massage or facial, book in for a consultation.

This book will not make you an aromatherapist but it will give you a basic understanding of this ancient art. It will inspire your aromatic appetite, prompting you to sniff out more information.

MEASURING INGREDIENTS

It is important that you measure the ingredients in your blends accurately. For this you will need a dropper (if a droplet cap is not fitted to the essential oil bottle), marked in amounts up to 1ml, a beaker, which will measure amounts greater than 1ml, and some metric measuring spoons for larger amounts. All these items can be purchased at a pharmacy.

Note that millilitres have been abbreviated to 'ml' and grams to 'g' throughout the book.

1ml	1 marked dropper	18–20 drops
2ml		36–40 drops
3ml		54–60 drops
4ml		72–80 drops
5ml	1 teaspoon	90–100 drops
10ml	2 teaspoons	
15ml	3 teaspoons (1 tablespoon)	
20ml	4 teaspoons	
25ml	5 teaspoons	
30ml	6 teaspoons	1 fl oz
40ml	8 teaspoons (2 tablespoons)	1⅓ fl oz
50ml	10 teaspoons	1⅔ fl oz
125ml	½ cup	4 fl oz
250ml	1 cup	8 fl oz
500ml (0.5 litre)	2 cups	16 fl oz
750ml	3 cups	24 fl oz
1 litre	4 cups	32 fl oz

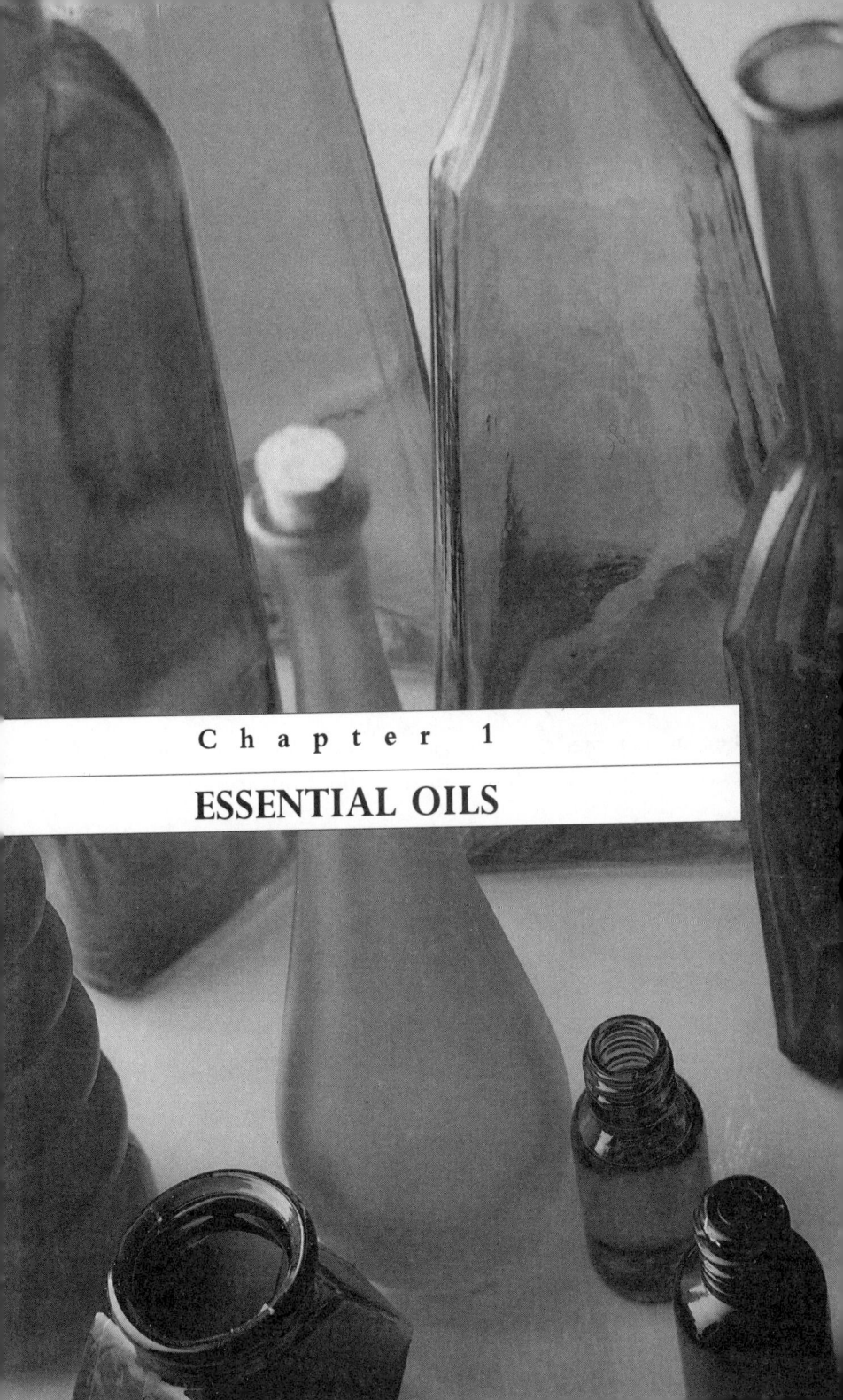

Chapter 1
ESSENTIAL OILS

We come across essential oils in day-to-day life, often without knowing it. When we peel an orange, the keen essential oils spray out at our face, and when we pass a jasmine vine, its alluring aroma alerts our nose to the fact that the oils are there. Essential oils are the volatile (highly flammable/evaporate quickly) components of a plant that are responsible for the plant's odour. They are just one of the many chemical components contained within a plant. Extracted from the flowers, roots, leaves, stems, bark, wood or seeds of selected plants, essential oils capture the secrets of a plant's vitality, long after the plant has perished.

> To prove the volatility of essential oils, squeeze an orange peel next to a candle flame and watch the sparks fly.

Let us explore the fascinating world of therapeutics and beauty that utilises these valuable gifts from nature.

MODERN AROMATHERAPY

Aromatherapy in modern times refers to the specific use of essential oils to influence positively the mind, emotions, body and soul. Its aim is to bring vitality and balance to each aspect of the human make-up. Various methods (massage, inhalation, compresses and so on) are used to achieve this and they will be discussed later in this chapter.

The term 'aromatherapy' was coined in 1928 by a French chemist, Dr Gattefossé, who was working in the family's perfumery business. One day he badly burnt his arm and, remembering that lavender was reported to heal burns, put his arm in a basin of lavender essential oil. The burn healed quickly, the result exceeding Gattefossé's expectations, and motivated him to embark on more research into essential oils. This classic tale is found in many aromatherapy books.

Another French professional, Dr Valnet, extended the therapeutic work of aromatherapy in medical and psychiatric disorders.

Marguerite Maury, an Australian beautician who married a French doctor, was also interested in aromatherapy and could see its potential in her beauty treatments. It was due to her initiatives that aromatherapy has developed as part of natural beauty regimes.

To find an ancient perspective we must travel back to the origins of botany and its use in perfumery, religion and healing.

ANCIENT BOTANICAL SNIPPETS

The origins of essential oils can be traced back to China, India and Egypt many thousands of years ago. It is known that in China, the *Yellow Emperor's Book of Internal Medicine* indicated the use of opium and ginger for therapeutic and religious purposes. In India the *Vedas*, the 'bible' of Ayurvedic medicine, written in the 7th Century BC, stipulates the use of aromatic plants such as sandalwood, cinnamon and coriander. Papyrus manuscripts of Egypt tell of aromatic gums and oils such as frankincense that were used in embalming, and of perfumes made for the Pharaohs and offered to the gods by the high priests.

Two Greek philosophers, Herodotus (482–425 BC) and Democritus (460–370 BC), visited Egypt and there recorded a wealth of information about perfumery and natural medicine. Another Greek who contributed much to the use of plants in healing was Hippocrates (c.460–377 or 359 BC). He is called the 'father of medicine' for his work in this area. Dioscorides, a first-century physician, is well known for his impressive work in listing 500 plants in *De materia medica*.

Distillation (a form of extracting essential oils from plants) was thought to be invented by an Arab philosopher and physician called Avicenna (980–1037 AD). However, a terracotta distillation unit, known to be from around 3000 BC, was uncovered in 1975 in a museum at the base of the Himalayas. Nonetheless, Avicenna wrote tens of books on the subject of plants and medicine.

Crusaders traded widely with a vast assortment of essential oils. They even kept their route a secret to safeguard the precious cargo. Perfumes from Arabia were much sought in Europe around the 13th century. At the time of the Black Death in Europe, aromatic plants were worn around the neck to combat the deadly plague. A German physician and alchemist, Paracelsus (1493–1541 AD), wrote a detailed book on medicine and in particular mentioned essential oils such as cedarwood, rose and sage for their therapeutic properties. His work was to become well known among physicians and pharmacists.

The great herbalist Nicholas Culpeper (1616-54 AD) advanced the therapeutic knowledge of herbs and essential oils into the 17th century.

HOW DO ESSENTIAL OILS WORK?

Used properly, essential oils work to heal and positively influences our emotions, mind, body and soul.

Skin Absorption

Essential oils have a small molecular structure, which allows them to be absorbed down through the layers of the skin (via the hair follicles, sweat glands and fat cells) until they reach the tiny blood capillaries and lymph vessels — their ticket to circulate throughout the body. A carrier such as a base oil has a larger molecular structure and is absorbed into the top few layers of skin only, where it nourishes and moisturises.

Lavender is the only essential oil that can be used neat on the skin. All other essential oils must be diluted in a carrier (a substance that transports essential oils into the body) such as air, water or oil.

Massage (my favourite) and compresses are the most effective methods of promoting absorption via the skin.

Inhalation

If I walk past freshly mown grass, I'm immediately transported back in time to the fun I use to have playing in the grass as a child. Smells can evoke emotional responses in people. This is how ...

There are a few theories on odour and how it can affect us. A popular theory is that there are millions of nasal receptors lining the nasal passages. Each receptor is individually shaped and will only receive an aroma that fits its shape. When the receptor and aroma are connected, they bond together in much the same way as a key in a lock. Once this is achieved a signal is sent to the limbic system (the emotion centre of the brain) and neurochemicals are released (via the nervous system) either to relax or to stimulate us.

Aromatherapy burners, lamp rings, steam bowls, tissues and potpourris are all effective means of inhalation. The quantity of essential oil that is actually absorbed by these methods is minute, as much of the oil is vaporised in the room. For a therapeutic effect, however, this tiny amount is more than sufficient to positively affect our system.

Now you know why inhaling orange oil or rose oil can make you feel so good.

Ingestion

Because of the small quantity of essential oil required for a therapeutic effect, ingestion is not advised without advice from an aromatherapist or a doctor qualified in aromatherapy. When essential oils are taken orally, most of the substance is directly absorbed and in this quantity can be toxic. In France, however, aromatherapists are doctors and they often prescribe highly controlled amounts of essential oils internally with good results.

How Much of the Essential Oil Is Absorbed?

In *The Aromatherapy Workbook* (Thorsons, 1993), Shirley Price gives the following approximate estimates for the amount of essential oil that may be absorbed while using aromatherapy in a day:

0.1 of a drop may be absorbed into your body from your aromatherapy skin care products;
0.01 of a drop may be absorbed from an aromatherapy burner or vaporiser;
0.5 of a drop may be absorbed during therapeutic use for a health problem.

By this, you can see how powerful essential oils can be. They can evoke therapeutic and pleasurable responses in minute quantities.

> ### French Ingenuity
>
> French aromatherapists treat an infection in a very practical way. They take a sample of the bacteria present and place it into several Petri dishes containing a range of highly antibacterial essential oils. They do not identify the bacteria by name (*E. coli*, *Staph. Strep.* and so on), but simply return to the Petri dishes 24 hours later and treat the patient with the essential oil that was most successful in killing the bacteria. What a good idea.

In Australia, the United Kingdom and United States, essential oils are used internally only sparingly, for example, one drop in honey or as a gargle. For the lay aromatherapy enthusiast, it is important never to experiment with internal use of essential oils.

EXTRACTION

Many factors can affect the quality and yield of the essential oils obtained from the flowers, twigs, wood, leaves and other parts of a plant. These include the species of plant, the soil conditions, the time of day the plant is harvested or gathered, the weather conditions and temperature during growing and harvesting, and the waiting period between harvest and extraction. For example, 1 tonne of lavender flower heads will yield 12 litres of essential oil, whereas 1 tonne of rose petals will yield a different amount. Lavender is left to dry for a few days before extraction, while fresh rose petals are processed as soon as possible. Whether or not each plant is grown and harvested under optimum conditions can mean the difference between a good essential oil producer and a mediocre one.

Expression

The essential oils contained within the rind of citrus (lime, lemon, bergamot, mandarin, tangerine, grapefruit, orange) fruits are extracted by this method. For economic reasons, citrus juice manufacturers usually express the oil as well. The citrus rinds are placed in a vice type of cold press and squeezed. A sponge below collects the essential oil. The sponges are then squeezed to extract the oil. The rinds were processed by hand originally, but the size of the industry today necessitates the use of machinery.

Essential oils extracted from organically grown citrus plants are obviously purer and more desirable than those that are not. They are also usually more expensive. Check with the supplier.

Expressing oil at home

You can express your own essential oils from the rinds of citrus fruit if you have access to large quantities of rinds. While this can be fun, it would not be practical if you were using the oil regularly.

Place the rinds in a small cold press and place a sponge underneath to catch the oil. Squeeze the sponge to retrieve the essential oil.

Distillation

The majority of oils (lavender, myrrh, sandalwood) are extracted by steam distillation.
1. Water is heated in a separate boiler to produce steam, which travels into a vat where the plant material is gathered on grills. In some situations the plant material is covered with water.
2. The steam causes the essential oils to evaporate and rise.
3. A cooling coil or pipe condenses the contents back into liquid form; that is, water and essential oils.
4. Depending on the density of an essential oil, it will

either float to the top of the water or sink to the bottom. It is then separated out by a strategically placed tap.

Distillation at home

If you are prepared to sacrifice an old pressure cooker, it will make the ideal distiller. However although this exercise is fun to do you do not obtain a great amount of essential oils.

Collect your plant material, using information from Chapter 9 as a guide. Half-fill the cooker with plant material and cover completely with water. Put the lid on and heat slowly.

Once steam begins to rise, fit a long plastic hose to the outlet valve and direct it to a collection container. Surround the plastic tube with a tea-towel filled with ice (or a few packets of frozen peas wrapped in a tea-towel).

As the steam rises from the cooker, it is condensed by the coldness of the ice, and the water and essential oils will trickle slowly into your container.

The steam should be maintained at a low level during the entire process.

ENFLEURAGE

Still used in France today, enfleurage is used to extract essential oils from delicate flowers such as jasmine and roses. It is a labour-intensive process and essential oils obtained from this method command very high prices.
1. Wood-framed glass sheets are covered with a purified animal fat such as lard.
2. Hundreds of hand-picked petals from the delicate flowers are placed on the lard. They are left for a day until their essential oils have been absorbed into the fat.
3. The petals are removed and fresh petals are placed over the now partially aromatic lard. This process is repeated several times until the lard has the required odour. It

usually takes several weeks. The scented fat is called a 'pomade'.

4. Pure alcohol (ethanol) is washed through the pomade to extract the essential oil, then a distillation process removes the alcohol. The resultant essential oil residue is called an 'absolute'.

Maceration

Maceration is used commercially to extract essential oils and other therapeutic properties from a limited number of plants such as calendula, carrot and hypericum. The plants are placed in a vegetable oil-filled vat and stirred for several days. The essential oils are drawn into the vegetable oil, then the liquid is filtered and ready for use.

Maceration at Home

Fill a preserving jar with flowers (jasmine, rose, calendula or others). Cover the plant material with a vegetable oil (almond or sunflower) and a small quantity of wheatgerm, the anti-oxidant-rich oil.

Place the jar in a warm area (a windowsill is ideal) and leave it for just over a week, gently shaking it occasionally.

Fit a muslin cloth or fine strainer over the opening of the jar and filter the substance. Hey presto! An inexpensive bath or massage oil.

Shopping for Essential Oils

The perfume and food industry are big users of synthetic or adulterated 'essential' oils, or 'non-essential oils' as I like to say. These oils are not used in aromatherapy. The synthetic copies lack the vitality that only nature can provide, and side-effects have been reported from their usage.

Oils can be tampered with in a number of ways: by adding alcohol, bulking a natural essential oil with a synthetic agent, substituting an odour-similar (not therapeutic-similar) oil for a more expensive oil, and extracting isolated ingredients such as terpenes from cheaper oils and adding these to another essential oil.

Synthetic and adulterated oils are cheaper and they give the perfume and food industry a consistent standard of oil.

Now you can see why it is crucial to buy essential oils from a reputable company. Some ways of checking that what you are buying is an essential oil and not a synthetic are discussed below. See also Buying Tips for each essential oil in Chapter 9.

BOTANICAL NAME

Make sure the essential oil you are about to purchase has a Latin or botanical name as well as a common name on the label. Otherwise you could be paying for an inferior-quality oil. Always be suspicious of an essential oil that has no botanical name on its label.

The best quality (and the most expensive) sandalwood to use for aromatherapy comes from Mysore in India. It is far more therapeutic and effective than its cousin from the west of India and even the Australian sandalwood. If you don't know the difference between them, you could be paying for a quality that just isn't there. But how can an aromatherapy beginner tell which one is which?

The answer is: by knowing the botanical or Latin name and even the origin of the essential oils you are interested in purchasing. For example, *Santalum album* originates in Mysore, whereas *Amyris balsamifera* originates in the west of India. Buyer beware! I have seen some bottles of sandalwood from western India selling at the price of the Mysore oil. The telltale sign is that there is no botanical name on the bottle and only tiny print on the side that says it is from western India.

Variation in Price

If the essential oils in a store vary in price, this is a good sign. Essential oils that are 100 per cent pure should vary in price. Orange oil (from the rind) will be priced at around $9 (Aus.) for 15ml whereas frankincense may be around $37 for the same quantity. So, I'm talking large differences in price in some cases.

The prices of essential oils vary so greatly because every plant has a different essential oil yield and availability. The less the yield, the more labour intensive the process of extracting the essential oil. The scarcity of a plant will affect the oil's price. Some oils may be expensive but they can last for two to three years or more, if stored correctly. Another consideration for your essential oil investment is that only small quantities are required to obtain good results.

If several varieties of so-called pure essential oils are all similar in price, it is highly unlikely they are pure. These oils are usually diluted with a base oil or they may contain synthetic oils. To obtain the best results with aromatherapy always use the real thing.

Dark-coloured Bottles

Essential oils are extremely volatile and sensitive to sunlight. Dark-coloured (amber or blue) bottles (fitted with a droplet dispenser or cap) are the best for storage of essential oils. If pure essential oils are stored in clear glass containers, walk past them as these oils will not last as long as the ones stored correctly.

At home, it is important to keep your oils out of sunlight. Some of the larger essential oil companies provide convenient wooden boxes in which to store the oils.

Gas-Liquid Chromatography (GLC) Testing

There are many constituents that are captured within an essential oil. A GLC is used by reputable companies to test the quantity and level of many of these known constituents. There are standard 'plates' of information that already exist for high therapeutic levels of the constituents contained in each oil. These plates are compared with the essential oil being tested. If there is a large variation between them, the oils should be rejected. Check with the in-store assistants where you buy good-quality essential oils; they should know if the manufacturer performs GLC testing.

Buying Essential Oils Checklist

➤ They have a botanical and common name on the label.

➤ They vary in price.

➤ They are stored in dark-coloured bottles.

➤ The essential oil supplier conducts GLC testing.

USING ESSENTIAL OILS

There are various ways in which you can use essential oils in aromatherapy to achieve your desired outcome. All involve the use of carriers for, as we have seen, all essential oils (except lavender) must be diluted in a carrier before being absorbed or inhaled. Carriers include air, as in steam inhalations or aromatherapy burners; water, as in baths; and oil, as in massage. They are an integral part of aromatherapy in action.

Outlined below are the basic tools that you will need to accompany essential oils to allow you the many beneficial experiences of aromatherapy. Each chapter of this book, including the summary charts in Chapter 9, will give you an abundance of aromatherapy blending recipes and ideas.

Note: It may be best to read Chapter 9 (after reading this chapter) to obtain more information on blending and essential oils. This will give more meaning to the terminology such as 'notes' and the recipes supplied.

Aromatherapy Burner or Vaporiser

Allowing pleasant vapours to waft in a room can be welcoming to a visitor or soothing to a tired mind and body. You can create the aromatic atmosphere in whichever room you are in.

An aromatherapy burner is a device (usually ceramic) that has a hollow section to hold a short candle and a dish above to house water and essential oils. Buying your burner from an aromatherapy manufacturer is recommended. The cheaper versions often leave too short a space between the candle and the bottom of the dish, causing the contents to boil.

After lighting the candle and filling the top dish with water, it's time to add your selection of essential oils. Three or four essential oils are usually used. In total, place up to 8 drops of your combination in the water. For example, if you want a relaxing blend of sandalwood, lavender and neroli (orange blossom), the ratio of drops may be 2:4:1, respectively. This can be derived from your aroma preference for an oil or by examining the blending factors and notes (see Chapter 9) of an essential oil.

Keep an eye on the water/essential oil level. It will need to be topped up every couple of hours.

Clean the dish out after use, using soapy, warm water and a cloth that has been put aside for this purpose only. If you don't clean it out, you will get a mishmash of odours that will interrupt the definite odour and therapeutic purpose of the newly chosen blend.

An electric vaporiser or diffuser is available that has a fan attached to help disperse the oils. This can be of particular benefit during convalescence of very young or old people. The electric vaporiser is quite expensive when compared with the non-electric version. Ask an aromatherapy manufacturer or stockist about it.

Method

➤ Choose an aromatherapy burner or vaporiser from a reputable aromatherapy products supplier.
Use up to 8 drops of essential oils in the water-filled dish, selected from up to three different essential oils.
Clean out the dish after use with warm, soapy water, then wipe clean.
➤ An electric vaporiser is available that can be of benefit during convalescence.

BATH

There's nothing better than a warm bath after a long day of 'busy-ness'. Aromatherapy can enhance the benefits you receive from soaking in a hot tub.

While the water is running add up to 8 drops of essential oils into the bath. Again, look at the blending factors and notes of the oils you choose. As with vaporisers, usually no more than three different blends make up the 8 drops. Do not be heavy-handed or add more than the 8 drops, otherwise you may come out of the bath with stinging legs! Believe me, I tried it one day with a blend of frankincense, lavender and bergamot. Ouch!

If you have bought a ready-made aromatherapy bath oil or you have made your own using essential oils and a base oil, around 5ml (1 teaspoon) is sufficient to add to the running water. Bath oils can be particularly useful if you have dry or scaly skin. While you inhale the wonderful vapours the oils will smooth and soften the skin.

You will need to clean the bath after each aromatherapy experience. A telltale ring around the bath will let you know. Clean with warm, soapy water or your regular cleaning agent.

Footbaths can be a quick way to relax and, you've probably guessed it, you add 8 drops of essential oils when you're filling a large foot tub. I love to put a handful of fresh rose petals in the water and massage the feet with a base oil to feel really pampered. You can massage yourself, but it always feels better when someone else does it for you.

Method
➤ Place up to 8 drops of essential oils in the bath or 5ml of a pre-prepared blend.
  Wash the bath after use with warm, soapy water or your regular cleaner.
➤ Use 8 drops of essential oils in a foot bath.

Beauty Treatment

See Chapter 8 for information on how to make your own aromatherapy natural beauty products.

Compress

A compress is a piece of cotton gauze that has been soaked in an essential oil/water mix. It is of particular use for reducing fever, relieving abdominal cramping and cystitis, and many other ailments.

The size of the area being treated will determine the number of drops of essential oils and amount of water used. As a guide for a large area such as the abdomen, place 8 drops of essential oils into half a litre of agitated water. Soak the gauze in the water, squeeze it and apply to the area.

There seems to be two schools of thought as to the length of time the gauze is applied: one suggests it should be changed after an hour while the other recommends an 'on and off' type of approach. I have found either to work well.

An aromatherapist may use other ingredients in a compress such as linseed wrapped in the essential oil gauze to draw out a boil.

Method
- Soak cotton gauze in essential oil/water mix; example, 8 drops of essential oils to 0.5 litre (16 fl oz) of water.
- Replace the compress after an hour or more often.

Douche

A douche is a water and essential oil rinse to a specific area. For example, a tea-tree oil douche can be beneficial during a bout of vaginal thrush. Add up to 6 drops of essential oils into a litre (32 fl oz) of warm water, agitate well. Squat in an empty bathtub and splash the mix into the affected area.

Method
- Use up to 6 drops of essential oils in 1 litre (32 fl oz) of water for a douche.

Lamp Ring

This is a small ring, usually made out of ceramic, that has a groove in it into which a few drops of essential oils are added. The ring is then placed over an upright light bulb in a lamp. The heat from the light bulb helps to dissipate the vapours throughout the room.

Be very careful not to spill essential oils onto the light bulb. They are volatile and may ignite.

Method
- Place 2–4 drops of essential oils onto a lamp ring. Take great care not to drop essential oils onto the light bulb.

Massage

Aromatherapy massage is one of the most luxurious forms of body therapies available, whether you're delighting in a facial or a full-body massage.

When you step into an aromatherapy clinic, you can truly leave the world behind you. You are greeted by relaxing music, welcoming blends of essential oils wafting from a burner and a friendly floral atmosphere.

After a short discussion the essential oils are selected for your body massage or facial.

Body massage

Aromatherapy massage combines the proven techniques of Swedish massage, Shiatsu, reflexology and Chinese therapies in its own unique style. As a naturopath I was taught Swedish, shiatsu and remedial massage. After learning the aromatherapy technique, I could not go back to using solely one of these techniques. The unique technique and the wonderful effects of the essential oils leave me, as well as the client, feeling good at the end of giving an aromatherapy treatment.

During the massage the body's meridians, or energy pathways, are followed and rebalanced. The massage movements help to stimulate lymphatic drainage (removing wastes from the body), are restorative to the nervous system (helping you to cope better with stress) and improve blood circulation (bringing nutrients to the tissues). Add to this the effects of vitality that essential oils can bring, and you will feel like new again!

During the massage the aromatherapist will be looking for any physical signs of congestion or imbalance in the body. These may be indicated by cold or hot spots, red blotches in certain areas or obvious musculo-skeletal peculiarities. The aromatherapist may recommend a referral to an osteopath, naturopath or an appropriate health practitioner.

Facial

An aromatherapy facial is a unique experience. The technique differs from that of a traditional beauty facial. With aromatherapy the neck, shoulders, scalp and face are massaged and pampered by a combination of gentle but firm aromatherapy movements. Natural cleansers, floral toners and an essential oil-rich massage cream replenish the skin. A steam — for example, a thyme steam to remove blackheads — or exfoliating treatment may also be given. I make my own fruit, flower and clay facial masques and individualise them to suit each skin type. While the masque is drying, your feet are revitalised with a massage and a hot lavender towel. One hour or an hour and a half later you usually need to be woken from your deeply relaxed state.

To ensure that you are being treated by a qualified aromatherapist, look for their diploma (not certificate) in aromatherapy, ask the practitioner where they trained and for how long, or ask if they are a member of an aromatherapy association.

Massage for the beginner

This book will give you aromatherapy recipe blends for massage and list contra-indications for the oils mentioned (see the 'Safety' notes for each oil, Chapter 9). However, only basic massage techniques are given. Please note that these are not aromatherapy techniques. I would not be doing the aromatherapy technique any justice by trying to condense it here. You could fill a book just discussing and teaching the technique. Look out for aromatherapy massage workshops or enrol in the aromatherapy diploma course for first-hand knowledge (which is always best when learning massage). When rubbing or massaging, make sure you have short, clean nails and that your hair is tied back.

In short, for a massage, add 1 drop of essential oil for every 2ml of base oil.

Base or Carrier Oils

The base or carrier oil is a vital partner of essential oils when applying aromatherapy massage. These nutritious and low odour oils assist to transport essential oils into the skin. Essential oils are too concentrated for the skin which welcomes these oils when they are diluted. Most base oils are derived from nuts or seeds and deliver unique healing properties of their own.

Choosing your base oil
(Available from health food stores or supermarkets)
Almond oil, sweet: One of the most widely used oils for face and body in aromatherapy (even though a little more expensive). It contains vitamin A, E and some B vitamins.
Apricot or peach kernel oil: Suitable for the whole body. It is high in essential fatty acids and some vitamin E (excellent skin healing properties).
Avocado oil: A rich oil that is high in vitamin E. Usually blended with other base oils to be used in dry skin conditions.
Jojoba oil or wax: A thick, highly stable liquid wax which is suitable for hair treatments or blended for body use.

Perfume

If you have a favourite essential oil or blend that you enjoy, why not use it as a perfume?

Put a drop of essential oil in 1ml of base oil and rub it into your pulse points, which are located on your wrists, behind your ears and at the back of your knees!

I love using a ready-bought dilution of 2 per cent damask rose oil in jojoba oil. You may wish to replenish your aromatherapy perfume dab every few hours. Remember, lavender is the only essential oil that can be applied neat to the skin.

Method
- Add 1 drop of essential oil to 1ml of base oil and place it on your pulse points (wrists, behind ears or knees).
- Ready-made dilutions of essential oils are great for this purpose.

POTPOURRIS, PILLOWS AND MORE

Essential oils lend themselves beautifully to enhancing the scent of rooms, closets, drawers or linen. Throughout this book, especially in Chapters 3, 4 and 5, you will discover the 'how to' of making your own potpourris, pillows and more.

I did read recently, however, that well-to-do European houses place scented tissue paper between the linen to keep them smelling fresh. What a good idea for refreshing well-worn sheets.

SPRAYS

Rid fleas, or make your own deodorant or room freshener with an aromatherapy spray. Plastic should not be used to house an aromatherapy mix. Use a glass or stainless-steel spray container (usually available from hardware or garden centres).

To a litre (32 fl oz) of filtered water add around 15–20 drops (in total) of essential oils. This will keep for 2–4 weeks before a fresh batch is required.

Method
- Place 15–20 drops of essential oils and a litre (32 fl oz) of filtered water in a stainless-steel or glass spray container.
- Keep for 2–4 weeks before making a fresh batch.

Steam Inhalation

Whether it's for a cold or flu, sinus or a beauty treatment, a steam inhalation can do wonders for clearing nasal passages and opening the pores.

Fill a medium-sized bowl with hot or boiling water. Add up to 6 drops (some people prefer 3 drops) of essential oils into the bowl. Place a towel over the head and slowly inhale. It is best to stay under the towel for a minute or two.

Method
➤ Add 3–6 drops of essential oils to a bowl of hot or boiling water. Drape a towel over your head, and inhale the vapours for a minute or two.

Swab

A swab is a therapeutic wipe of an area. It can be used in the case of an insect bite, a graze or haemorrhoids.

Place 6 drops of essential oils in 125ml of water (4 fl oz), dunk a cottonwool ball into the mix and squeeze it to remove excess liquid. Gently wipe over the affected area.

Method
➤ Place 6 drops of essential oils in 125ml (4 fl oz) of water. Dunk a cottonwool ball into the liquid, squeeze and gently wipe over the affected area.

Tissue

A few drops of an essential oil on a tissue, handkerchief or cottonwool ball can give you a quick and easy inhalation of essential oils. You will need to add more essential oils after an hour or so.

Method
Place a few drops of essential oils onto a tissue or cottonwool ball to receive a quick and easy essential oil benefit.

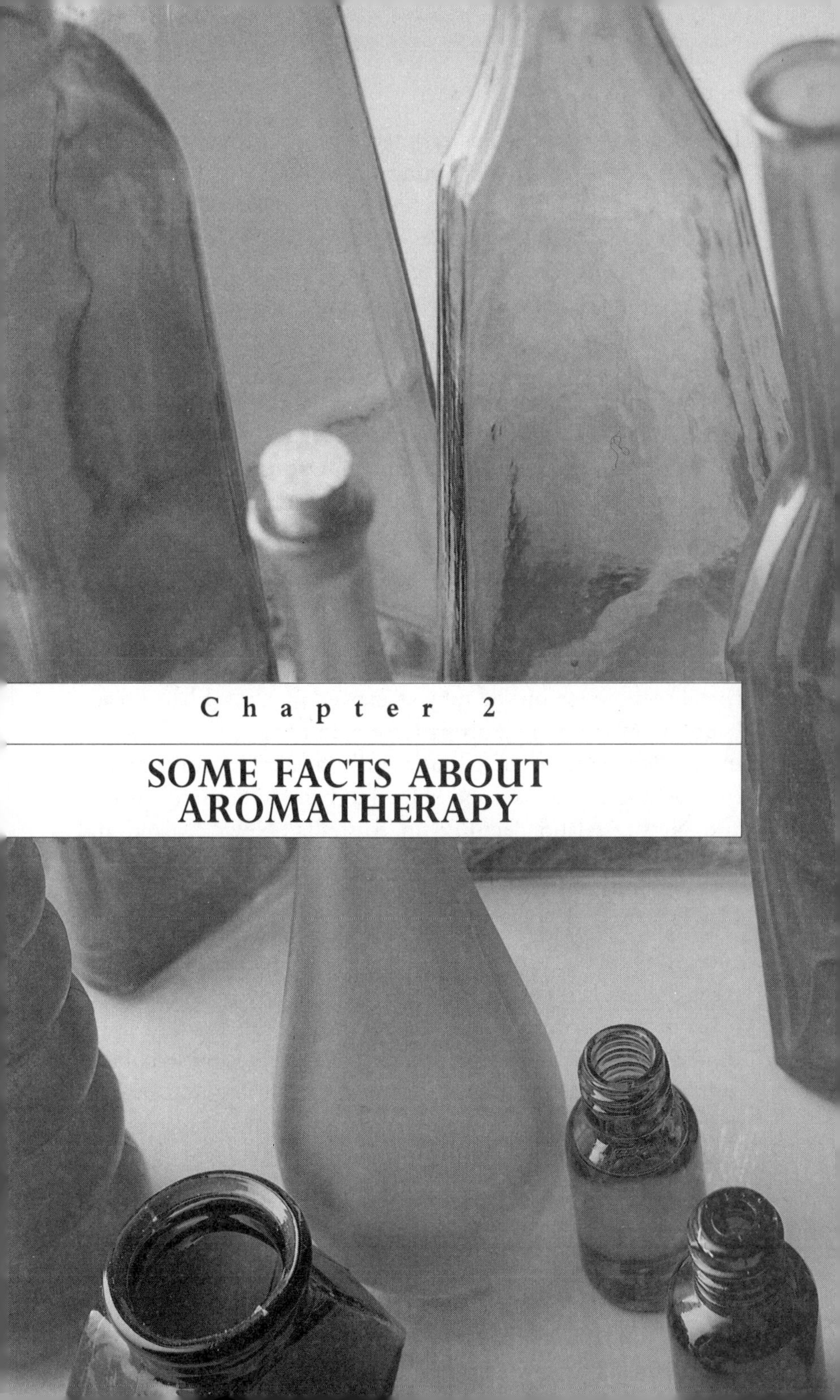

Chapter 2

SOME FACTS ABOUT AROMATHERAPY

I'll share with you in this chapter my personal aromatherapy regime, details about becoming an aromatherapist, what to expect in a consultation and some information on the areas in community health where aromatherapists are becoming more involved. Let me first tell you about my discovery and journey into the world of aromatherapy.

Have you ever experienced those goose-flesh type of tingles that seem to accompany a 'right place, right time' or a 'this is where I'm meant to be' situation? Usually it's by trusting and following your intuition or gut feeling that you land in this wonderfully fulfilling position. I'd heard about aromatherapy and decided to investigate a course. Upon receiving the information I promptly enrolled. During my aromatherapy studies those goosy flesh things were working overtime. I became 'hooked' on aromatherapy, and I knew it was about to become a big part of my life.

I was so impressed that I booked myself into an international conference on the subject, started practise (I had already been in practise as a naturopath for a number of years), assisted in the formulation of commercially available aromatherapy (pre-blended) products and helped to launch them in Australia and New Zealand, lectured in Australia, New Zealand and Malaysia, ran workshops, gave television and newspaper interviews and wrote an outline for this book!

I have found that when you know what you want in life and are prepared to put in the hard work to steer you in the right direction, the opportunities seem to appear magically in front of you. After drafting an outline for this book, I mentioned to a few close friends that I wanted to write it but I didn't approach any publishers at this time. A few months after completing the outline I received a call, asking me if I would be interested in writing a book on 'Aromatherapy'! As you can imagine, the word 'yes' torpedoed out of my mouth.

A DAY IN THE LIFE OF AN AROMATHERAPIST

I incorporate aromatherapy into my day by using essential oils in my washing and beauty routines, during my meditation or yoga exercises, and around the house to set a mood in a room or to disinfect areas. And of course I use them at work in my clinic rooms. Even in 'my other life' as a freelance public relations health consultant, I use aromatherapy. The essential oils help to clear my mind when brainstorming or writing communication strategies, and they help to relax me and boost my confidence when making a presentation to a client.

The essential oils that I use personally and in the clinic come from reputable suppliers. Brands include Springfields, InEssence, Jurlique and a 'practitioner-only' brand called Aromatherapie. While I was in the United Kingdom I was impressed by the Tisserand and Shirley Price essential oil range.

Now back to my aromatherapy day...

Morning

Accompanied by soft music (I love Japanese flute music), I do yoga exercises (for 20 minutes) or a meditation while the calming orange, lavender and sandalwood essential oils rise from an aromatherapy burner.

Next I take a shower, using soap containing sandalwood or rose essential oil and a skin brush. If I have a big day ahead, I'll use an energising shower gel containing lemongrass, rosemary and patchouli to get me going.

After the shower, I apply an aromatherapy body lotion, tone my face with either the lavender or neroli toner and apply the easily pre-prepared aromatherapy moisturising cream to my skin (see beauty recipes in Chapter 8). Then I apply (to the back of my wrists) an aromatherapy perfume of sandalwood and orange or an appropriate oil to meet the mental or emotional needs of the day (see Chapter 5).

To Work

If I'm working from home, that usually means I'm writing, so a blend of rosemary, basil and lemon burns merrily away in the vaporiser. It keeps my concentration focused on the job at hand.

If it's a clinic day, I benefit from the essential oils that I use on my clients. Whether it's a naturopathic or aromatherapy session, the aromatherapy burner is always on. I can honestly say that I've never finished a clinic day feeling drained. Sometimes a little tired (depending on the number of clients), but never drained.

If I've been out and arrive home in the afternoon, I may give Honey, my gorgeous cat, an aromatherapy 'de-fleaing' treatment (see Chapter 3), which she strongly dislikes.

I usually carry a first-aid kit of tea-tree, lavender and peppermint, a small quantity of base oil and cottonwool with me wherever I go. This can provide quick relief in any of life's little emergencies, such as grazes, headaches, nausea, heartburn and so on (see 'Holidays', Chapter 6).

My friends and family are occasionally treated to aromatherapy massages and home-made aromatherapy gifts. A foot or shoulder massage seems to be the order of the day.

Night

At night, I really love to pamper myself. If I'm having a bath, I will usually add a teaspoonful of a self-made bath oil, which comprises of fresh jasmine flowers or rose petals (see 'Maceration', Chapter 1). While I'm soaking I'll apply a fruit and green or pink clay masque to deeply cleanse my skin.

My nightly facial treatment consists of cleansing and toning (the same as the morning) and I also use a nourishing face oil. This rejuvenating blend (see Chapter 8) contains apricot kernel oil, evening primrose oil and a little wheatgerm oil. To this I add the 'youthful complexion' essential oils of neroli, lavender and rose. I wake up looking 10 years younger ... well, almost.

If there's romance in the air, read Chapter 5. I've given away a few secrets there!

Please don't be overwhelmed by the amount of aromatherapy that can be used in one day. In reality, some of the situations mentioned above would happen weekly or longer apart. I've mentioned as many examples as possible to show you how aromatherapy can be incorporated into your life.

But more now on how to become a qualified aromatherapist and what to expect from an aromatherapy consultation.

HOW TO BECOME AN AROMATHERAPIST

A budding aromatherapist participates in a one-year full-time or two-year part-time course. If you have already studied anatomy, physiology and massage as part of a diploma course, as have naturopaths, masseurs and beauticians, for instance, you can enrol in a post-graduate course, which involves around 120 hours of aromatherapy study. Either way, it's interesting, stimulating and hard work! Your local aromatherapy association will be able to point you in the direction of a registered school.

The course covers the history of essential oils, their chemistry and how they interact together and with medication. It includes an intensive investigation of 20 (or more) essential oils, discussing any hazards associated with their use, and their cosmetic and therapeutic usages. It covers case histories, diet and lifestyle. The course also looks at setting up a clinic and the 'code of ethics'. Around 60 hours (in the post-graduate course) is spent learning and perfecting the unique aromatherapy massage and facial techniques. A basic first-aid certificate has also been introduced as a requisite.

Aromatherapists quite often do further study in the chemistry of essential oils and counselling.

The investment in essential oils is quite a substantial one for a practitioner. My essential oil dispensary would be valued at around $2000–3000 (Aus.). This includes the more expensive oils such as rose, neroli, and chamomile, and the essential oils contained in the larger 'practitioner-only' bottles. The towels, blankets, pillows, massage bed, burners, base oils and creams, natural aromatherapy beauty products or ingredients if you make your own come on top of that. If you are a beginner, don't be alarmed; it will probably cost you well under $100 to get started with half a dozen low to moderately priced essential oils.

Your 'Aromatherapist': Fact or Fiction?

Masseurs, beauticians or other practitioners who have attended a weekend or short course are not aromatherapists. In many locations I have seen these untrained practitioners advertising aromatherapy treatments when, in fact, they are merely using a small selection of essential oils in with their regular massage technique. This can be misleading or even potentially detrimental for the client.

The consumers are not getting what they are paying for, as they are not being massaged by the unique aromatherapy technique. They can unwittingly be harmed by a treatment given by someone who lacks a comprehensive knowledge of essential oils. These practitioners do not have the background in chemistry and pharmacology needed to know and understand the reactions between certain medications and essential oils, or their contra-indications. In other words, they don't know when to use essential oils and when not to.

Always look for an Aromatherapy Diploma on the wall or

ask the practitioner where they were trained and for how long. Are they a member of an organisation such as the International Federation of Aromatherapists, which only accepts therapists as members who have completed the full training?

AROMATHERAPY TREATMENTS: WHAT TO EXPECT

When you go to an aromatherapist there are a number of treatments from which to choose. You might select a one-hour full-body massage (including a mini facial), a one-and-a-half hour full-body massage and facial (including masques), a facial, or a back and foot massage. This list may vary slightly among practitioners.

An aromatherapist is interested in your whole well-being. During an initial consultation, the first 10 minutes will be spent in gathering information from you, the client. After finding out what you are there for ... a relaxing massage, a sore lower back or another health problem ... the therapist will ask questions about your medical and family history: Who is your doctor or regular health practitioner? Are you taking any medications or supplements? Have you had any surgery? What illnesses have you suffered? Are there any hereditary illnesses in your family? Do you have high blood pressure, epilepsy or are you pregnant (some essential oils are contra-indicated for these conditions)? The aromatherapist might also ask for information about your diet and lifestyle, and will do a skin analysis to assess accurately your facial skin type.

The aromatherapist will skilfully select essential oils and base oils that are suited to your physical, emotional or mental needs. There will be different oils for the face and body. An aromatherapist is trained not only to give you a relaxing massage but to blend essential oils to assist in the healing of numerous health conditions such as cystitis, arthritis, migraines, psoriasis, thrush and bronchitis.

The therapist will ask you to smell the essential oils selected (usually no more than three in a blend) and will then tell you why they were chosen. It is important that you find the blend aromatically pleasing; if you don't, say so and others will be chosen. The aromatherapist will leave the room and allow you to disrobe in private. A towel or gown is provided and you lie face down on the table. On returning to the room, the practitioner will cover you more and make you comfortable.

Your individualised treatment begins (see 'Massage', Chapter 1). At the end of the treatment you will be supported to a sitting position and given a drink of filtered water or herbal tea. The practitioner will leave the room to allow you to dress. I like to give clients a small sample of the massage oil or facial masque I have used so that they can enjoy using them at home. A teaspoonful of the massage oil will complement the next bath.

Some people have weekly, monthly or bi-monthly treatments. If you are seeking treatment for an ailment, regular sessions are necessary in the short term.

WHAT WILL MY DOCTOR SAY?

Not all doctors are open to, or have knowledge of, the benefits of aromatherapy and healing. However, in France, aromatherapy is acknowledged and widely used by doctors. Contact between the aromatherapist and the local GP is encouraged, as it leads to a better understanding between the two practitioners. An aromatherapist will consult with your doctor concerning the proposed treatment of a serious medical condition.

Many nurses who are trained aromatherapists are using aromatherapy to varying degrees for home- and hospital-care patients. In this case the nurse obtains consent from the patient, their doctor and the nursing manager. Having said that, more and more non-nursing aromatherapists are working within hospitals, especially in the maternity sections (see the section on pregnancy, Chapter 5) and in centres for the disabled.

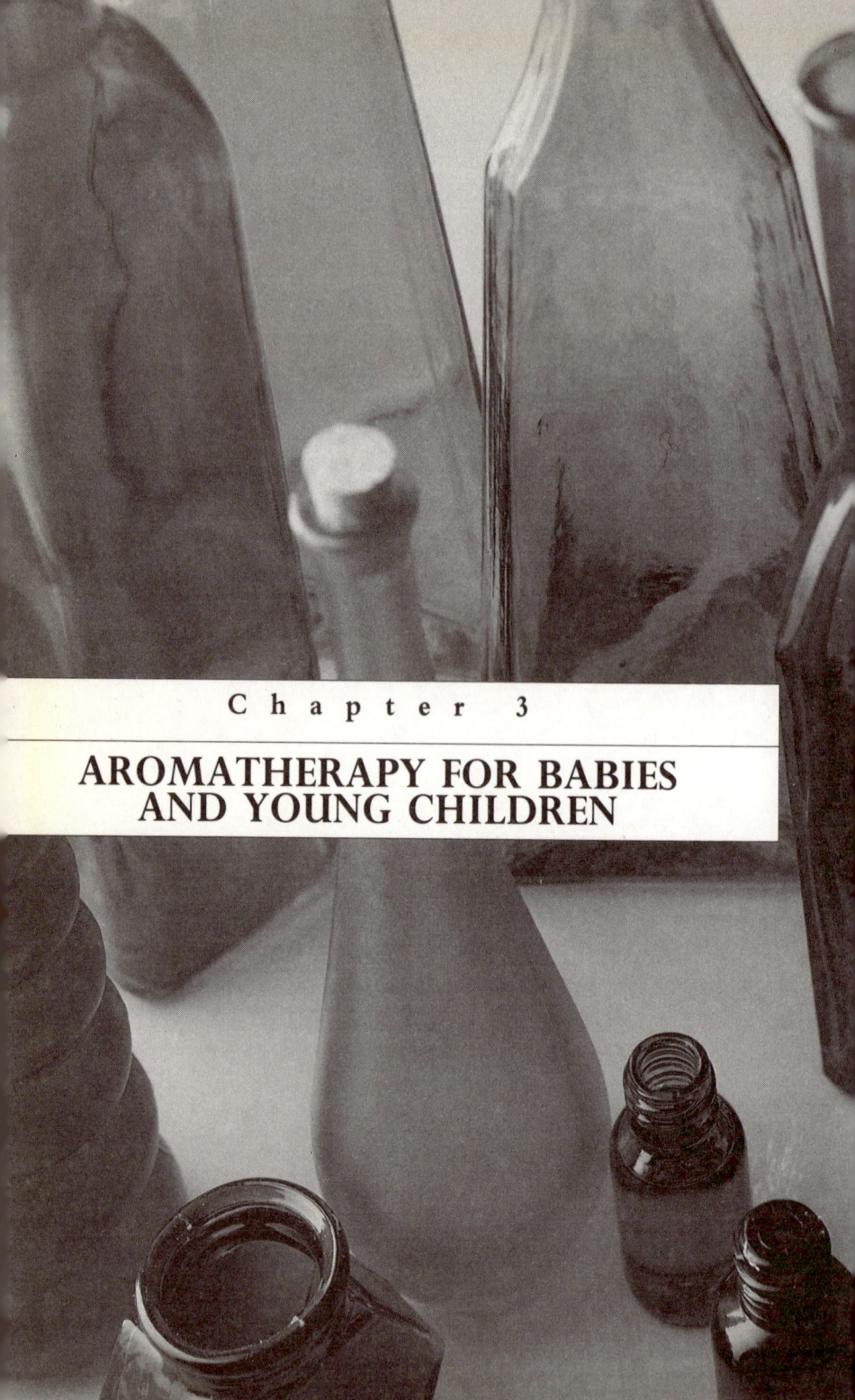

Chapter 3

AROMATHERAPY FOR BABIES AND YOUNG CHILDREN

The excited anticipation of upcoming events and the energy and exuberance of a child at play can tempt a warm smile from even the 'Mr Scrooges' of this world. Children are great teachers. They are sparkling reminders that can awaken the sometimes dormant 'fun' in adults.

Children love the ritual that can accompany special occasions. Like leaving a tooth-filled sachet for that famous fairy or writing to Santa and leaving him out some goodies to enjoy. Aromatherapy can enhance these rituals and touch the lives of children in many different ways.

Aromatherapy for the special 'events' in children's lives, for common childhood ailments and for massage for under 12 years will be covered in this chapter.

NOTE: ADULT SUPERVISION IS REQUIRED WHEN USING ESSENTIAL OILS. ESSENTIAL OILS CAN BE TOXIC IF SWALLOWED.

AROMATHERAPY AND IMPORTANT OCCASIONS

TOOTH FAIRY, 'COME TO ME'

The tooth fairy loves lavender oil, and if 1 drop is placed on a tooth that is surrounded by cottonwool and tucked under a pillow, it will attract this rare visitor.

FIRST DAY OF SCHOOL JITTERS!

Fear of the unknown is normal. Ask the school bullies if they were nervous on their first day and they'll secretly tell you that their knees were knocking too.

To relax and calm your child (well enough to enjoy this historic day), place 1 or 2 drops of orange essential oil onto the corner of a handkerchief or tissue. Ask the child to take regular sniffs. It's also useful for parents.

Bathtime

Great! In go the toys, the bubbles and, of course, that nice-smelling stuff. 'They think I'm in here to get clean (oh, that 'clean' word shouldn't be in the dictionary). This is my play-time.' A soap containing essential oils or a bubble bath will add joy to a child's bathtime, while satisfying the primary objective of washing them.

Add 2–4 drops in total of essential oils to a child's bath. Lavender is a good choice.

Special Occasion Insomnia

When the excitement of a special occasion (for me it was a school excursion or a birthday party) just won't let your child get to sleep, reach for the lavender pillow.

You can make a pillow by placing the dried flower heads of this light purple beauty into a drawstring bag and adding 3 drops of lavender essential oil. Inhaling the sleep pillow regularly will allow for pleasant dreams ...

Heavenly Bedtime Comfort

Children find comfort in knowing their guardian angel is around to help watch over their family and friends. Angels adore the sweet smell of jasmine or rose. To help in communicating with these special heavenly friends, place some of these flowers or their essential oils into a water-filled bowl beside the child's bed. You never know, the flutter of wings just may be heard.

Present for Grandma

Mum, spare one of your old, clean pantyhose (the more colourful, the better). Fill the cut foot section with drops of Grandma's favourite essential oils mixed with a potpourri of dried flowers. Tie with a ribbon attached to your child's personalised tag to Granny. I hope you've already guessed — it's a fragrant drawer ball.

Happy Birthday

Boys may not be amenable to that 'sweet smelly stuff' but when they grow up they'll find essential oils spread throughout their toiletries. The more 'masculine-smelling' essential oils are cypress, sandalwood, lemon, cedarwood, pine and juniper. Gifts scented with these oils such as a car-shaped sandalwood soap certainly won't get tossed aside.

For the birthday girl, well, tell me when to stop! An aromatherapy blend of 2 drops of orange and 3 drops of lavender in 20ml (⅔ fl oz) of apricot kernel oil placed in an elegant perfume bottle (dolly will appreciate a dab also) will bring hours of sophisticated delight. Aromatherapy flower-, fairy- or heart-shaped soaps or hair-care products are great gifts with an embroidered handtowel. Or you could make an aromatherapy herbal sachet to dangle from a padded hanger or a pressed-flower birthday card with a drop of a sweet-smelling pure essential oil on the back of it. Pure essential oils should not leave a mark on the paper whereas synthetic or adulterated oils will.

Homework, Here We Come

Yes, you read the heading correctly. While essential oils cannot lead a child by the arm into the much dreaded homework position, they can motivate and clear the mind to improve concentration.

It's well worth investing in an aromatherapy burner. Fill the top container with water, add 2 drops of lemon and 3 drops of rosemary, light the candle below and watch the brain cells spark.

For exam nerves, burning neroli and lavender can calm mild anxiety.

Pets

You know the story — the child gets the pet, but who looks after it? That's right, Mum or Dad. Kittens and puppies are gorgeous and quite often little Johnny or Mary will play with them in the house. This can be fun, but what about fleas? Aromatherapy can be used to de-flea your pets. (Garlic can too, if you regularly place a capsule or tablet in their food.)

Add 2 drops of tea-tree and eucalyptus and 3 drops of lavender essential oil to your pet's shampoo and separately to the rinsing water. Add a more concentrated blend to a bottle of water and spray it around the pet's bed.

Some Aromatherapy Hints

➤ Place an aromatherapy lamp ring on a child's night light. (Take care not to spill any on the bulb.) Place a few drops of lavender or marjoram oil (mild sedatives) on the ring to help the child sleep.

➤ A drop of rosemary on a bookmark, kept nearby when the child is reading, will improve retention.

➤ Place potpourri pillows with a few drops of your child's favourite essential oils in the wardrobe, beside teddy, under the pillow or on a mobile.

➤ Soak a child's sports socks (especially the footy ones) in a basin of warm water with several drops of peppermint essential oil to remove unpleasant odours.

➤ A hyperactive or overly energetic child can be calmed by placing 2 drops of vetiver, the 'tranquillity' essential oil, with 3 of lavender in an aromatherapy burner. Place the burner in the child's room (out of reach) or place 1 drop of the essential oils in a little base oil and rub this onto the pulse points.

➤ Christenings or special religious events can be blessed and enriched by burning frankincense or myrrh around the child.

AROMATHERAPY AND COMMON CHILDHOOD AILMENTS

Now you can include aromatherapy essential oils in your family's natural medicine chest. Essential oils can be used singly or as an adjunct to other remedies such as vitamins, minerals, homoeopathics or herbals. Aromatherapy can be used therapeutically to treat acute and chronic illness. However, if an illness is serious in nature, you should naturally seek the advice of a health practitioner.

BABIES

Studies are now validating that babies use their sense of smell to identify their mother. Babies can discriminate between their mother's odour and another mother's odour. There is even suggestion that smell plays an important role in the bonding process and that a mother's smell can help to calm a baby.

If you would like to use an essential oil as a signature for your baby, it is best to use a calming one such as lavender, neroli or sandalwood (the latter two in with a base oil). Be careful not to be too heavy-handed with the amount you place on your pulse points. After telling a friend about these findings she liberally splashed lavender on herself as her signature. When she placed six-month-old Tim beside her, the wince and the surprised 'you pong' look he gave her told her to reduce the amount of lavender she used. I'm told he has been calmer since she started using lavender.

On a more serious note, neglected war orphans have been nurtured back to health with the help of an aromatherapy signature. Practitioners in one study used roman chamomile (for its soothing and sedative qualities) and lavender (for its calming and uplifting qualities) to combat the greatest barrier of these children ... the fear of being touched. Because of their signature smells, used in conjunction with puppets and a signature tune, the children began to trust the adults and started along the road to recovery.

Following are aromatherapy treatments for common baby ailments.

Colic

Spasmodic contractions of the intestines causing a build-up of gas and tension, and affecting babies up to three months of age. The baby may draw the legs up towards the chest during a spasm. Colic often follows rushed or tense feeding times. It may also be caused by an allergy to milk.

Aroma aid: Gently massage the baby's stomach with a blend of one drop of lavender or chamomile with 6ml of a base oil such as apricot kernel oil.

Cradle cap

Overactive sweat glands can cause a yellow/brown crust on the scalp. Dead skin cells and oil can build up in crusty patches in babies with very oily skin.

Aroma aid: Add 3 drops of lavender to 20ml (⅔ fl oz) of apricot kernel oil and carefully massage this over the crusty area. Repeat daily.

Crying

Research is now showing that a mother who responds quickly to her child's crying during the early months will have a baby who cries significantly less in the coming months. The quick response time helps to build a trusting relationship between mother and child.

Some of the reasons for a baby's cry include hunger, pain or colic, wet or soiled nappy, loneliness, boredom, overtiredness or overstimulation. And sometimes, no matter what you do, nothing will alleviate the crying.

Crying: Ryan's Story

Ryan, aged six months, like most babies, cries a lot. His mother came to see me in frustration, stating that once all the obvious causes had been eliminated, he still kept crying. Naturally, there are many mothers who are drained of energy by interrupted sleep, caring for a child's needs, household chores and, for some, part-time study or work. Kathy was no exception and desperately needed a solution to her problem.

Kathy is studying by correspondence and attends residentials at the university. She has great support from her family but Ryan usually travels with Kathy at these times. A baby's constant cry is obviously not desirable in dormitories or during lectures.

Treatment

I suggested to Kathy that she use a few drops of neat lavender on her pulse points, put a drop in Ryan's bath and massage a few drops into him with a blend of apricot kernel oil every second day.

Kathy's results were very positive. On commencement of the use of lavender, Kathy noticed that Ryan cried much less and seemed calmer.

> *I couldn't believe how quickly it worked. One night while we were away on campus, Ryan began to cry. Feeling self-conscious about waking the other students (the walls were paper-thin), I immediately rushed for the lavender bottle and put the drops on myself and Ryan. Almost instantly he calmed down and didn't stir again that night!*

Kathy also reported feeling more energetic and relaxed.

Nappy rash

A red, inflamed area of skin around the buttocks that can be caused by wet or dirty nappies and allergies. To avoid nappy rash, keep the baby clean and dry as much as possible. Wash in the creases of skin and pat dry, rather than rub, with a towel. Some people even suggest blow-drying your baby's bottom after a bath!

Aroma aid: Mix 2 drops of bergamot and 1 drop of lavender in 20ml (⅔ fl oz) of apricot kernel oil. This can be gently wiped or dabbed over the sensitive area at each nappy change, helping to reduce inflammation and heal the skin.

Sunburn

A baby's skin is very sensitive to sunlight, and is also much thinner than an adult's and more vulnerable to the effects of ultraviolet light. Many experts say that a child under the age of two should not be exposed to the sun for more than 10 minutes. A hat, cotton shirt and the regular application of sunscreen are essential when baby is in the sun. In spite of all the awareness about care in the sun, babies are still being hospitalised each year with sunburn.

Aroma aid: For mild sunburn, place a few drops of lavender into a small portion of aloe vera gel. Gently apply this to the area using cottonwool.

Teething

At around five or six months of age a baby may start to teethe. The lower two teeth usually precede the upper two. Your baby may dribble excessively, seem irritable, have a rash on one cheek and go off food.

Aroma aid: Place a drop of chamomile into 5ml of apricot kernel oil. Massage generally over the body daily. Remember, once into the circulation the chamomile can target the teeth, helping to reduce the pain and calm the child. If you find the essential oil too expensive, a homoeopathic chamomile remedy is also beneficial (and much cheaper).

Young Children

Abrasions
Minor wounds where the surface of the skin has been grazed.
Aroma aid: Place 4–6 drops of tea-tree oil in 125ml (4 fl oz) of water. Immerse a cottonwool bud or ball into the mixture, squeeze and gently apply over the wound's surface.

Asthma
Widespread narrowing of airways, wheezing and coughing with difficulty in breathing are the characteristics of asthma. It is most commonly triggered by an allergic reaction, infection or emotional stress.
Aroma aid: Use a drop of lavender and peppermint (along with frankincense if you can afford it) in a steam inhalation 2 or more times per week ... depending on the severity of the asthma. If a steam inhalation is 'too much' for the asthmatic, remove the towel and allow the child to breathe from the bowl. Using these oils in an aromatherapy room burner regularly is also recommended.

Bed-wetting
An involuntary release of urine during sleep, which can be prompted by emotional or nervous factors or by a urinary tract infection.
Aroma aid: If the bed-wetting is emotional or nervous in origin, to relax and calm the child, use 5 drops of bergamot and lavender in 40ml (1⅓ fl oz) massage oil or add a few drops of each to a tissue to inhale. For an older child (8–12yrs) add 2 more drops each of the oils to the abdominal massage blend.

Bee sting
After a bee has stung, it is important to leave the stinger attached to the person. By pulling it out, you release further venom into the wound.

Aroma aid: Apply neat lavender to the sting area. Alternatively, apply mildly diluted tea-tree oil. Detach the stinger with tweezers after several minutes.

Bronchitis

Acute bronchitis is caused by bacterial or viral invasion and is characterised by coughing, yellow/green-coloured mucous and spasm of the bronchial area (narrowing of the air passages).

Aroma aid: Use the same oils as for asthma in a steam inhalation two or three times daily to relieve congestion and coughing.

Bruising

A usually superficial, bluish-purple area found beneath unbroken skin.

Aroma aid: As well as homoeopathic Arnica drops taken internally, a must for bruising, the essential oil of lavender, applied neat or with fennel on a cold flannel or cotton compress, is recommended. They will help to decrease a bruise's usual seven-day stay.

Burns

First-degree burns: reddening of the skin without blistering. Second-degree burns: blistering of the first two layers of skin. Third-degree burns: destruction of the full thickness of skin and can involve fat, muscle and bone.

Aroma aid: See the case study below. Lavender applied neat, in a massage oil or placed in an aromatherapy burner is suggested.

Burns: Ciaran's Story

On 15 January 1994, Ciaran, aged two, was badly burnt in a house fire. The hospital assessment of Ciaran's condition was recorded as 'Superficial burns to the face; more severe to the head; severe to the hands; also has blisters over his shoulders'. Ciaran's plastic surgeon was amazed at his speedy recovery. He stated that children with burn injuries such as Ciaran's usually take two to three months longer to heal than his short few weeks. The answer for this accelerated healing was aromatherapy.

Having already used essential oils since her pregnancy, Mandy, Ciaran's mother, knew she wanted to help her son with aromatherapy. After receiving advice from local aromatherapists she went about her treatment with the agreement of the hospital staff.

Using lavender and other carefully administered essential oils Ciaran's burns were treated over a period of weeks. Ciaran underwent a skin-graft for his right hand. It was treated with a mixture of healing essential oils after the operation, which proved so successful that the plastic surgeon was amazed by the rate of his recovery.

Ciaran was discharged just three and a half weeks after his admission to hospital. Ciaran's parents continue to apply the aromatherapy treatment.

The burn to Ciaran's forehead is still evident and he has a few scabs and small patches on his head where the hair did not regrow. His right hand, which was grafted, requires regular massage to maintain its suppleness and to straighten his fingers. His left hand has fully recovered.

Catarrh

An inflammation of a mucous membrane, usually of the nose and throat, causing excessive secretion of thick phlegm or mucus.

> ### Chronic Catarrh: Lucy's Story
>
> Lucy, aged two, had suffered from thick green catarrh since eating solid food. She experienced ear infections and her eyes would 'stick' together. She was given antibiotics by her doctor.
>
> Already in her short life, her adenoids had been removed, her sinuses drained and grommets (used to help drain fluid from ear drums) fitted into her ears. The aromatherapist treating Lucy noted that despite all of her health problems Lucy had a quiet and happy nature. The mother was shown how to massage her chest with an aromatherapy blend of sandalwood, lavender and lemon at home.
>
> Although after a few weeks no permanent improvement had been observed the treatment of light massage was persevered with. The Aromatherapist began to suspect that food allergies were involved and Lucy was taken off milk and wheat. Steam inhalation was used to loosen the catarrh and Lucy's mother was shown how to massage her chest with essential oils at home. Within a few days there was a dramatic improvement.
>
> Lucy has remained almost completely free of catarrh and has had no need of further antibiotics.

Chickenpox

An acute contagious disease caused by the varicella-zoster virus, and is characterised by fever and skin eruptions. The incubation period is 11-24 days.

Aroma aid: Add 4 drops of lavender to a hand bath and gently wash the child with a flannel. Use lemon, tea-tree and lavender in an aromatherapy burner.

Colds and flu
Viral infections of the respiratory tract characterised by sneezing, nasal discharge and malaise.
Aroma aid: Regular steam inhalations with a few drops of tea-tree, eucalyptus and lemon relieve congestion. Eucalyptus and tea-tree can be placed on a tissue and inhaled regularly. To prevent the spread of the virus to others at home, it is recommended that you burn these essential oils in a room burner.

Earache
Pain in the ear, usually caused by infection.
Aroma aid: Mullein oil is my first choice. (This is usually available in ready-to-use form. Follow the directions on the label.)

Fever
The normal oral body temperature is 37°C (98.6°F). When this rises by 1°C, a person is said to have a fever.
Aroma aid: Place 2 drops of rosemary and 2 drops of tea-tree in a basin of cold water. Swish a cotton flannel in the aromatherapy water mixture, squeeze and place on the child's head. Repeat at regular intervals.

Lice
Small parasitic insects that attach themselves to the hair and clothing of humans. It is a highly contagious condition.
Aroma aid: After washing the hair, rinse the hair, especially the roots, with a mixture of 10 drops of lavender in 500ml (16 fl oz) of water. This can be mixed and shaken in a spray bottle. Repeat regularly.

Measles
A contagious viral illness marked by red spots on the skin, inflammation of the respiratory mucous membrane and fever.
Aroma aid: Add 1 drop of thyme or pine, 1 drop of tea-tree and 3 drops of lavender into a basin of warm water, and gently sponge the body with the mixture. Use a few drops of lemon, eucalyptus and pine in an aromatherapy burner.

Mumps
A contagious viral disease characterised by fever, headache and vomiting, which often precedes the swelling of one or more salivary glands.
Aroma aid: Use the essential oils in the aromatherapy burner as per measles. Carefully massage (with warm hands) the glands with a mixture of 2 drops of tea-tree and 3 drops of lavender in 20ml (⅔ fl oz) of a base oil. Repeat at regular intervals.

Tonsillitis
Inflammation of a tonsil or tonsils caused by a bacterial or viral infection.
Aroma aid: A steam inhalation with a few drops of tea-tree and thyme and 1 drop of lemongrass, repeated 2 or 3 times daily, is recommended.

Warts
Small horny outgrowths on the skin, usually of viral origin. They occur singly or in clusters.
Aroma aid: Add 1 drop of lemon and tea-tree oil to a dressing and change every day for a fortnight. And tell the warts to go away. It worked for me and I had 20 warts on my hands as a child!

Whooping cough
An acute contagious disease caused by an infection of the mucous membranes of the airways by the bacteria *Bordetella pertussis*.

Aroma aid: A steam inhalation of a few drops of eucalyptus, tea-tree and lemon 2 or 3 times daily can relieve the coughing.

TEACHERS TAKE NOTE!

Aromatherapy is being used increasingly by teachers around the world to introduce harmony and motivation back into the classroom. I am receiving very encouraging feedback from colleagues and teachers participating in my workshops who report that not only were the pupils calmer and happier (after the use of aromatherapy) but their attention span also seemed to increase.

This feedback is suggesting that neroli, bergamot, lavender, chamomile and rose (used in an aromatherapy burner) are most effective in reducing hyperactive and aggressive behaviour. Sandalwood and vetiver also help to relax these pupils.

Other teachers are using eucalyptus, lemon and tea-tree in the burner during winter months when colds and flu are prevalent. This 'anti-bug' blend helps to discourage the spread of these debilitating ailments.

AROMATHERAPY FOR DEAF, BLIND AND MUTE CHILDREN

In the unseen or silent world of the sight- or hearing-impaired child, aromatherapy can offer a welcome channel of communication.

There are many heartening examples of aromatherapy helping the sensory deprived. Here are two cases that highlight the positive influence aromatherapy can exert.

Jim's Story

Jim had Down's syndrome and only partial sight in one eye. At 20 years of age his attention span was short and he experienced chronic sinusitis, constipation and dandruff.

He was put on a course of aromatherapy treatments which, over six months, yielded remarkable improvements. He began to enjoy his full-body massage and his concentration span improved steadily. The massage also quietened the aggressive behaviour which had previously been a problem area for him. Abdominal massage with essential oils eliminated his constipation, whilst inhalations cleared up his sinusitis. A scalp massage with tea-tree oil greatly improved his dandruff.

George's Story

George, aged 21, was profoundly deaf and blind, suffered from epilepsy, had aggressive and self-abusive tendencies, would not allow himself to be touched by other people and didn't wear clothes or shoes.

At first he was introduced to the smell of essential oils. Later touching in the form of massage was begun on a very gradual basis. In time he actively began to enjoy the massage and would make his way unaided to the treatment room and prepare himself for it. His aggressiveness was reduced and he began to wear clothes and explore the world around him. He now communicates through finger spelling.

In both cases aromatherapy seems to have had a profound effect in bringing the sensory deprived out of themselves, and allowing them to enjoy and look for external stimulation.

CHILDREN AND MASSAGE

Forget about pleading with your partner for that much-needed rub. Children are terrific and willing masseurs. They give wonderful shoulder, hand and feet massages and they love it when you reciprocate.

Outside of loving hugs our children don't receive a lot of nurturing touch. Healthy touch is a way of reassuring children that they are wanted and basically okay as human beings. Psychologists are now saying that children who are deprived of touch when they are young can be low in confidence and self-esteem as they grow up. So, gentle massages can be another healthy way of saying 'I care and I love you'.

Children's Massage Blend

As a general rule when massaging children, because of their smaller frame, reduce the essential oil dose.

6–12 years: One-half the adult dose★
2–6 years: One-third the adult dose
Babies: One-quarter the adult dose

★ The adult dose is as follows: for every 2ml of base oil use 1 drop of essential oil. So, if mixing 20ml (⅔ fl oz) of base oil, use 5 drops of essential oils for an eight-year-old child, 3–4 drops for a four year old and 1–2 drops for a baby.

Easy 8-step Foot Massage

Peppermint is refreshing while lavender will help to relax tired feet. As an adult dosage guide, place 4 drops of peppermint and 6 drops of lavender into 20ml (⅔ fl oz) of a base oil such as grape seed, apricot kernel or sweet almond oil.

The technique described below is easy for both children and adults to enjoy. It's probably a good idea to practise on your child first and teach them the basics.

1. Place two chairs facing each other or face each other on the floor. Rest the foot on a towel-covered leg. If a heavy adult's foot is too much for a child, place it on a towel-covered stool.
2. Apply the aromatherapy blend to the foot. Use sweeping movements with both hands up and down the foot. If tickling is a problem, use a firmer movement. A game of 'Round and round the mulberry bush' can be fun.
3. Next, slide the thumbs from the heel of the foot to the base of the toes. The thumbs face each other and slide away from themselves for this technique. Repeat this movement three times.
4. Again, make a few sweeping movements over the foot.
5. Do gentle toe lifts by placing the thumb at the base of the big toe and the fingers (lead by the index finger) on the other side of the toe. And, you guessed it, squeeze and travel up and off the toe. Repeat this on all toes.
6. Make some more sweeping movements over the foot.
7. Now make circular thumb movements from the heel to the toes. The thumbs are placed facing each other (as in the thumb slides) and small circles are made by the thumbs as they travel up the sole of the foot.
8. Finish with some light strokes over the foot and begin to massage the other foot.

This technique can be duplicated on the hands. Lemon or geranium can be pleasant essential oils (combined with a base oil) for the hands.

Easy Head And Shoulder Massage

Logistics need to be explained here. If a child is giving an adult this massage, they will need to sit on a chair or couch

while the adult sits on the floor in front of them. Lying on a towel on the floor is another option.
1. Before applying an aromatherapy blend, start by massaging the head from the base of the skull to the top of the head. Small circular movements feel great. A few gentle circular rubs on the temples can also be relaxing. Use slow movements and repeat each step 3 times.
2. Apply the oil with sweeping movements over the shoulders and up the neck.
3. Place the hands on each shoulder. Gently squeeze the shoulder muscles between the thumb and fingers. Repeat this over the shoulder area, then, resting one hand on the left shoulder, use the same technique with the other hand to massage the neck.
4. Repeat the broad, sweeping movements over the neck and shoulders.
5. Place the thumbs on either side of the spine and, with small circular movements, travel up the centre of the back until you reach the base of the neck.
6. Repeat the head massage and finish with light strokes down the back.

BABY MASSAGE

Babies adore massage. Because of a baby's size, the range of essential oils that can be used is limited, but tangerine, lavender, chamomile and rose are all safe.

Place 1 drop of the essential oil into 5–10ml of apricot kernel oil (my favourite base oil for babies). Please beware of using a mineral oil 'baby oil' on your child. They do not allow the skin to breathe. Natural is certainly better here. Light, gentle strokes over their body can be comforting and nurturing to a little babe.

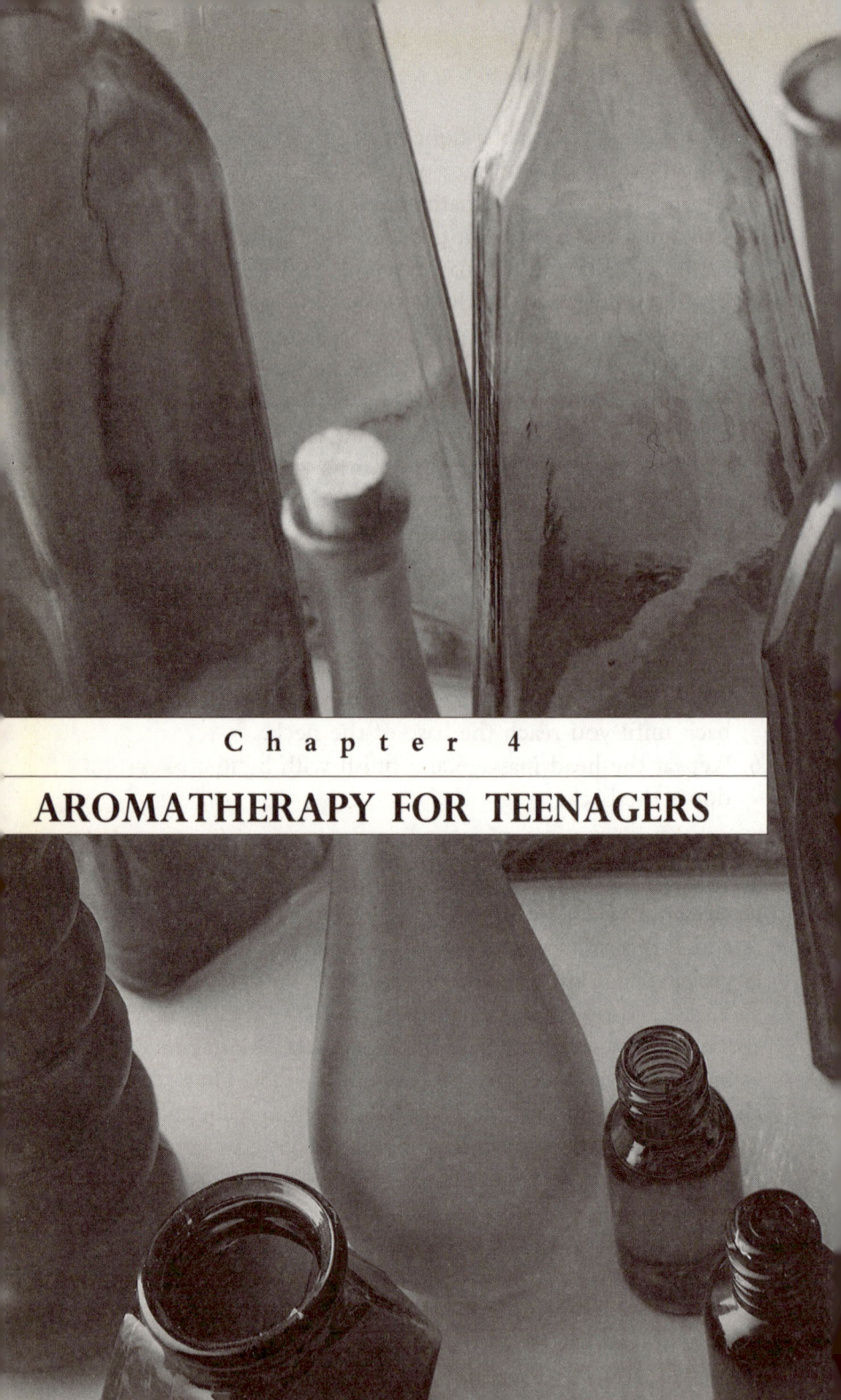

Chapter 4
AROMATHERAPY FOR TEENAGERS

Teenage years can be filled with fun and adventure. Suddenly you're allowed to do so many more things: going out — without Mum and Dad, learning to drive, dating. For some of you, though, these years may not be breezy in the emotional and physical departments. The pituitary gland makes sure of that as it works overtime releasing sex hormones that alter what you look like and how you feel.

Adolescence can in some cases mean conflict in family relationships. Teenagers may want to make decisions for themselves but find that they are hindered, because they are legally or financially dependent on their parents. It is a time when approval is sought more from peers than from parents.

Parents too must alter the way they are relating to their daughters and sons. Altering the old dominant parent–child pattern of communication to include adult–adult interactions can help to reduce conflict and improve the relationship.

Aromatherapy can help at this stage of life, rebalancing the mind, emotions and body. And just as well, because there's a lot to contend with. Acne, growing pains, premenstrual syndrome, cystitis, thrush, weight gain and more may be experienced physically, while mood swings, stress (peer-group pressure, exams), anxiety, internalising problems, low self-esteem and low self-confidence may be present emotionally. Aromatherapy can be a healing, uplifting and calming tool if used wisely throughout the journey of adolescence.

AROMATHERAPY AND TEENAGERS

STUDY

If only I had known about rosemary, basil and lemongrass as I crammed for geography and maths! The basic elements for success in learning are motivation and concentration. These essential oils are of paramount importance to the student. Rosemary and basil improve concentration and memory, while lemongrass energises and motivates tired (or unwilling) brain cells.

Place 4 drops of rosemary, 2 of basil and 2 of lemongrass in a water-filled aromatherapy burner. Position the burner on your study desk and take a few deep inhalations before commencing study. Experts recommend a 5–10 minute break from study every hour or two. Your burner will need to be topped up with water and more of the same essential oils after a few hours.

One study at the University of Cincinnati showed that students exposed to peppermint and lily-of-the-valley outperformed the control group (breathing unscented air) in repetitive tasks. Another showed that people who were exposed to lavender experienced less tension when working long hours on computers compared with those who were not exposed to the scent.

Exam Nerves

Well, you've got the information in your head but your tummy's in a flutter with all those butterflies. Aromatherapy is an excellent adjunct to calming exercises such as meditation or nutrients such as B-complex vitamins.

Place 2 drops of lavender and 4 of bergamot onto the corner of a tissue and inhale at regular intervals. Guys, if the thought of this blend sounds too floral, place 4 drops of cedarwood on a tissue for a similar, yet more masculine-smelling, effect.

These oils can also be blended into 10ml of a base oil and rubbed into the pulse points.

> ## MASSAGE AND TEENS
>
> Regular anti-stress aromatherapy massages are ideal for pressured teenagers. A massage gift-voucher once each month, or weekly during exam periods, will help to show them you understand the stress they are going through.

FIRST SHAVE

Let aromatherapy take the sting out of this momentous occasion by using a lavender pre-shave face soak.

Place a few drops of lavender into a warm basin of water. Dunk a washer into the mix, squeeze and apply to the area to be shaved for about 20 seconds or so.

DRIVER'S LICENCE

All I remember from my driving test is the astonishment I had at the uncontrollable shaking of my non-confident hands and legs ... not to mention embarrassment. Even the reassurance of my driving instructors went astray.

For confidence and calm, rub 1 drop of vetiver (dilute it in a few millilitres of base oil), the tranquillity essential oil, into your solar plexus (just between the lower ribs). Applying any of the anti-stress essential oil/base oil blends already mentioned (bergamot, lavender, sandalwood, cedarwood) onto your pulse points every two hours will help to calm your anxiety.

BOY MEETS GIRL OR VICE VERSA

Whether you're 15 or 45 a first date can be full of nervous excitement. So you need something to calm you and to help you enjoy the big date.

Neroli is expensive in its pure state but can be purchased already diluted in a base oil. Dab this uplifting and relaxing essential oil onto your wrist and behind the ears prior to your date. Or inhale it from a burner prior to leaving.

Broken Romance

See 'Relationship Endings', Chapter 5.

Rebellion

Conflict is inevitable in life. When our wants and needs are different from those of the people around us, impatience and anger can result. Often things are said that we later regret.

Geranium can help to ground you and to integrate your thoughts, while rose is one of the key essential oils that assists in dissipating anger. Placing 5 drops of geranium and 2 of rose in a water-filled aromatherapy burner is recommended.

Suicidal Thoughts

A sad fact is that Australia has a very high incidence of male teenage suicide. Teenagers usually talk only to their peers about the contemplation of taking their own life. The warning signs can be talking about suicide, deep depression, a feeling of hopelessness, giving away cherished possessions and getting affairs in order. Counselling is imperative to mending this situation.

Aromatherapy can be part of the solution. Particular essential oils are mild anti-depressants that can gently persuade you back to feeling good again. Or at least good enough for you to seek help from the appropriate sources.

Lavender (4 drops), bergamot (5 drops) and clary sage (3 drops) placed in a water-filled aromatherapy burner and inhaled at regular intervals will help to alter your state of mind to a lighter one.

Your Room Potpourri

Making a potpourri for your room can be fun and easy. And you'll know what has gone into it. Some of the ready-made ones are rife with synthetic aromas. Potpourris make inexpensive gifts for family and friends, too.

In the morning as soon as the dew has dried on the flowers, go on your picking spree. Half-open buds will retain their fragrance and colour longer than those in full bloom. Be as adventurous as you like with colour and odour.

Line a cardboard box or shoe box with paper. Spread the flowers evenly on the paper, then place the box, uncovered, in a warm, airy place for 10 days. Turn the flowers once daily during this time.

Place the flowers in a bowl and add 1 tablespoon each of orris root (available from a health food store or pharmacy) and salt to preserve the fragrance. Add a few drops of your favourite essential oils.

Put your potpourri in a lidded glass jar and open it for one hour each day to release the aroma in your room.

Summer Breeze

Mix together: 20 dried lavender heads, 12 dried red roses, the petals from 1 dried geranium, the orris root and salt, and 1–2 drops of each flower's essential oil.

Mystic East

Mix together: 12 dried roses, 3 lavender heads, 1 tablespoon of crushed and dried orange peel, 1 teaspoon of ground nutmeg and allspice, 12 whole cloves, the orris root and salt, and the desired essential oils.

AROMATHERAPY AND COMMON TEENAGE COMPLAINTS

ACNE

Acne is an inflammatory disorder of the oil-secreting sebaceous glands that is characterised by blackheads and pus-filled pimples. It can affect the face, back and chest. Cysts and scarring can occur in severe cases. Although the cause of acne is unknown, the steroidal hormone (androgens) is linked with acne.

Some teenagers are (regrettably, in my opinion) placed on long-term antibiotic treatment or told benzoyl peroxide lotion is their only hope. The greasy junk food that they are eating has not been disallowed and scanty washing instructions are given in some cases. It's a real pity because natural therapies, especially the antibacterial essential oils and sensible eating habits, have much to offer acne sufferers.

As acne affects the lives of so many teenagers, an in-depth view of the aromatherapy research and treatment will be presented here.

ACNE RESEARCH

The following study was conducted to see whether tea-tree oil is more effective than benzoyl peroxide (Basset et al. 1990).

The Department of Dermatology at the Royal Prince Alfred Hospital in Camperdown (NSW), headed by Professor Ross Barneston, performed a single blind, randomised clinical trial comparison study on 124 patients with mild to moderate acne. This study evaluated the efficacy and skin tolerance of 5 per cent tea-tree oil gel compared with 5 per cent benzoyl peroxide.

Method

Patients (60 females and 64 males), the mean age of whom was 19.7 years in a range of 12–35 years, were selected in accordance with the following criteria:
- They were free from intercurrent disease.
- They had not used or taken systemic antibiotics, steroids, retinoids, anticonvulsants or androgens in the 30 days prior to the start of the trial.
- They had not undergone topical acne therapy within two weeks of the trial's start.
- The females had not commenced or ceased the oral contraceptive pill in the six months prior to starting the trial.
- The males were without beards or moustaches.

Two groups were randomly selected. All treatments (5 per cent tea-tree oil, 5 per cent benzoyl peroxide) were packaged in identical sealed containers and stored in identical numbered boxes. Even though tea-tree oil has a strong odour, no patient was 'officially informed' as to which treatment they were using.

The patients were assessed initially and reassessed three times at monthly intervals. All assessments were performed by the same investigator.

The parameters used to assess the efficacy of each treatment over the period of their use were the number of inflamed lesions (superficial and deep) and the number of non-inflamed lesions (open and closed comedones). Oiliness, erythema, scaling, pruritus and dryness (graded 0 – nil to 3 – severe) were assessed to determine the skin tolerance.

Results

The results of this study showed that both 5 per cent tea-tree oil and 5 per cent benzoyl peroxide had a significant effect in ameliorating the patients' acne by reducing the number of inflamed and non-inflamed lesions (open and closed comedones), although the onset of action in the case of tea-tree oil was slower. Encouragingly, patients treated with tea-tree oil experienced fewer side-effects.

In the 'Discussion' section of this paper it was noted that tea-tree oil was better tolerated by facial skin. As well as the initial irritant effects of benzoyl peroxide, skin scaling, dryness and pruritus were among the side-effects experienced by patients in the trial. It was also suggested that using a higher concentration of tea-tree oil (as anecdotal use sees successes of concentrations up to 100 per cent) may speed its activity and the healing of acne.

Acne: Peter's Story

Peter, aged 15 years, came to me after trying popular acne treatments on the market to no avail. His acne presented with pustules on both the cheeks, blackheads on his forehead and large, blind pimples on his shoulders and upper back area. He was understandably embarrassed about his appearance and seemed quite introverted.

Treatment

Aromatherapy routine: morning and night
1. Wash with an essential tea-tree oil-based soap (Thursday Plantation or Blackmores offer therapeutic soaps) or an antibacterial face wash that is based on tea-tree oil. Pat the skin dry with a clean towel or tissue.
2. Use the following essential oil blend directly onto the pimples.

Base oil: 45ml (1½ fl oz) of apricot kernel oil (high in anti-inflammatory essential fatty acids that are important for healthy skin), 5ml of wheatgerm oil (high in scar-fighting vitamin E) and 10 drops of carrot oil (high in the good skin vitamin A).

An aromatherapy base cream can be used if you do not want to use the oil.

Essential oil: To the base oil add 12 drops of tea-tree, 8 drops of thyme and 5 drops of lemon.

3. Once or twice weekly, place 6–10 drops of the above anti-acne blend into a bowl of steaming water, put a towel over your head and stay over the bowl for 1 – 2 minutes. Keep your head around 30cm (12in) away from the basin. It is best to keep your hair clean and tied away from the back and face. For girls, make-up should also be kept to a minimum. And the big one — don't touch your face. To extract blackheads (don't touch the pimples) either use a special extractor that can be purchased from a pharmacy or gently squeeze the blackhead with tissue-wrapped index fingers. Dab the spot with the anti-acne blend after extraction.

Diet and lifestyle

Peter was given a sample daily diet, which consisted mainly of:
- 2–4 pieces of both fruit and vegetables.
- 2 servings of wholemeal foods (wholemeal breads, pasta, cereals).
- 1 serving of lean proteins (grilled fish, chicken with the skin removed, lean red meat, or pulses).
- 1 teaspoon of vegetable fat (use olive oil in cooking) or low-fat dairy.
- 6 glasses of purified water, the first of which contained half a squeeze of lemon to assist the detoxifying process.

The primary problem with acne is that the inflammation furnishes a cosy environment for bacteria to flourish. It makes sense, then, to decrease or eliminate for a time foods that promote inflammation and deplete the immune system, such as high portions of sugar and saturated fat.

Exercise improves circulation and the transport of oxygen and nutrients to the skin. Peter was asked to walk (or do an exercise he enjoyed) for 20 minutes 3 times per week and gradually double this over a four-week period.

Herbal help

Cleansing the inside of the body is also strongly recommended. If the person has been on antibiotics (they can wipe out the balance of favourable gut flora), a course of *lactobacillus acidophilus* is strongly suggested. A herbal tablet that assists in cleansing, improving the immune system and healing the skin was used once daily for Peter. The tablet is available from health food stores or pharmacies and contains the antibacterial herbs echinacea and calendula, with skin-healing zinc and vitamin A.

Results

After one month on this regime, Peter's face and shoulders had cleared dramatically. He was then instructed to use the anti-acne blend every second day and an oil-free moisturiser in between. It is important to note that when your body is in 'cleansing mode' through supplementation and diet, the skin may appear to be worse as the toxins are thrown out onto the skin. This usually calms in a week or so. Beware: if you eat chocolate or chips during this time, they will show up on your skin as pimples very quickly.

Other Teenage Complaints

Constipation

Irregular bowel movements or difficulty in passing faeces constitutes constipation. Therapists (especially naturopaths) intently ask questions to somewhat bewildered patients about their bowel motions. 'Do they float? How often are they? What colour are they?' Believe it or not, you can tell much about a person's health from the answers to these questions. For example, if the movement comes out in hard pellets, stress is usually the cause; if it is yellow in colour, the person has poor fat digestion, and so on.

Constipation is of particular concern with teenagers. If they suffer from pimples or acne, constipation will tend to make the condition worse as toxins build in the body. Natural remedies are best. Teenage diets are often low in fibre foods such as fresh fruits, vegetables and complex carbohydrates. Introducing these into the diet is a first step.

Aroma aid: A gentle abdominal massage using marjoram, lavender and rosemary often relaxes the area within minutes, with a normal bowel movement following the next day. To 20ml (⅔ fl oz) of sweet almond oil add 2 drops of rosemary, 3 of marjoram and 5 of lavender. If flatulence or diarrhoea is a problem, an abdominal massage using chamomile (1 drop), fennel (4 drops) and lavender (5 drops) is recommended in 20ml (⅔ fl oz) of base oil.

Cystitis

An infection of the urinary tract causing inflammation of the bladder. Burning urine, frequency of urination and, in severe cases, cramplike pain in the lower abdomen and blood in the urine can result. Females are more prone to cystitis because their urethra is short and bacteria can easily travel to the bladder. This condition is rare in males because their urethra is longer.

Aroma aid: Make a warm compress using 3 drops of bergamot, 3 of lavender and 2 of sandalwood in half a litre of warm water. Change when the compress cools, and repeat.

Additionally these oils can be added to a full bath or hipbath. Continue both treatments until the symptoms subside. For urethritis, substitute tea-tree oil for sandalwood.

Other: To reduce inflammation and acidity of the urine, add 1 flat teaspoon of sodium bicarbonate to a lemon barley drink (one glass bi-hourly for six hours). Avoid sugar, meat, shellfish, alcohol, tea and coffee. A tea of the herbs buchu, uva ursi and couch grass (available at health food stores) and 1–2g of vitamin C daily can also assist healing.

Glandular fever

An infectious illness that affects the lymph nodes in the neck, armpits and groin. The Epstein-Barr virus is responsible for the swelling, tenderness, fever, headache, sore throat and loss of appetite. Glandular fever has an incubation period of around a week.

Aroma aid: Unfortunately, I've seen many Higher School Certificate hopes dashed by the onset of this debilitating and long-lasting virus. Aromatherapy and other natural therapies can do much to shorten the duration of glandular fever.

Carefully massage the neck and affected glands with the following aromatherapy blend 2 or 3 times daily: 2 drops of lemon and tea-tree with 3 of juniper in 10ml of sweet almond oil. This is detoxifying, antiviral and helps to decrease any stress. Using the essential oils in a water-filled aromatherapy burner daily is also recommended. Sniffs of bergamot or bitter orange can help to lift the spirits.

Other: A diet low in sugar (including alcohol) and fats is strongly recommended. A naturopath can help with a herbal remedy of echinacea, cleavers, poke root and wild indigo to support the lymphatic system.

Herpes

Inflammation of the skin caused by a herpes virus. Type 1, or herpes simplex, is the common cold sore. It manifests as blisters around the lips. Type 2, or genital herpes, is sexually transmitted and, as its name suggests, appears on the genitals. Depending on the site of initial infection, cold sores or genital herpes can be caused by either type 1 or 2 virus.

Aroma aid: For type 1, apply a ready-made concentrated tea-tree oil-based cream onto the cold sore with a cotton bud. Alternatively, make your own antiviral blend by adding 5 drops of tea-tree oil to 10ml of base oil.

For type 2, add 5 drops of tea-tree oil to 10ml of warm water. Gently dab or wipe the affected genital area with a squeezed cottonwool ball that has been soaked in the blend. This needs to be repeated 2 or 3 times daily.

Other: The amino acid L-lysine is the main nutrient useful for treating herpes, although vitamin C, zinc and vitamin A can all be healing. Look for a tablet in your health food store.

Premenstrual syndrome

Most women experience physical and emotional changes during a normal menstrual cycle. But for some females, the changes occurring in the second half of their cycle can be distressing. The theories vary as to what causes PMS, but the popular belief is that the fluid retention, tender breasts, migraines, depression, backaches, lethargy and other symptoms are caused by diet, hormones and stress. It's a good idea to keep a menstrual diary for four months to see what symptoms are predominant.

Aroma aid: Add the following essential oils — sage (8 drops), lavender (12 drops), chamomile (5 drops) — to 50ml (1⅔ fl oz) of sweet almond or apricot kernel oil. Massage the oil around the lower back and ovaries daily around 10 days prior to the onset of the period, and place 10 drops in a bath.

MAKE YOUR OWN MENSTRUAL BLEND

Personalise your own menstrual blend using the chart below as a guide (see 'Blending' Chapter 9).

Symptom	Essential oil
Painful cramping	Bergamot, chamomile, marjoram, cypress, clary sage, sage
Fluid retention	Juniper, cypress, sage
Mood swings / depression	Bergamot, geranium, damask rose, lavender
Headache	Lavender
Lack of menstruation	Sage, clary sage, marjoram, myrrh
Excessive bleeding	Damask rose, cypress, chamomile

Premenstrual Syndrome: Megan's Story

Megan (14) started her period when she was 13 years old and since then had had increasing difficulties with her period — severe cramping pain, depression and excessive bleeding. The first two symptoms presented up to four days prior to her period, which was regular. She would not attend school for two or more days during this time.

Treatment

Megan was given a blend of cypress (12 drops), damask rose (5 drops), chamomile (7 drops) in 50ml (1⅔ fl oz) of apricot kernel oil. She was instructed to massage it onto her ovaries once weekly and then once or twice daily, one week prior to her period. And to place 10 drops of the blend in a bath. Megan was also asked to keep a diary on her symptoms.

A diet high in saturated fats (animal fats, full-cream dairy products, fatty meats) can increase the unfavourable prostaglandins in the body that increase inflammation, cramping and pain. On the other hand, a diet high in vegetable fats will promote the favourable prostaglandins that help to reduce these symptoms. This is one reason evening primrose oil is beneficial as it also helps promote favourable prostaglandins. The saturated fats in Megan's diet were reduced, along with sweets, fizzy drinks, alcohol, cakes, biscuits and chocolates, at least 10 days prior to her period.

One theory is that women crave chocolate around menstrual time because it is high in magnesium. Thankfully, many PMS formulations contain magnesium.

Additional supplementation for Megan included 1000mg of evening primrose oil 3 times daily, 10 days prior to her period.

Megan's initial visit to me was four days prior to her next period. The treatment commenced at this time. She noted that the symptoms slightly abated during her first period but noticed most improvement during the second month of treatment. The bleeding had noticeably reduced, and she was using only three pads, instead of five, each day. The depression had cleared and the cramping had stopped and she experienced only slight pain on the day prior to the period. All symptoms were absent during the third and following months.

Psoriasis

The skin cells multiply quickly in this common skin condition, which is characterised by patches of thickened, red, scaly skin. It affects five to 25 year olds, and twice as many girls are affected as boys, although this evens out nearer to adulthood. Hereditary, infection (onset often occurs up to 10 days after infection) and emotional stress can cause the symptoms to manifest or make them worse.

Psoriasis: Helen's Story

Helen, aged 16, came to me after suffering from psoriasis since the age of seven. Helen's mother also suffered from psoriasis as a teenager. Helen's neck, elbows and back were the most affected. She had noticed that her skin appeared worse around exam time and when there was tension in the house, such as arguments. She had been using a cortisone-based cream for several years. Having heard about the side-effects of this long-term treatment, she was seeking a natural alternative.

Treatment

Saturated fats, caffeine and sugar were reduced in her diet. She was encouraged to eat healthy skin foods such as carrots, pumpkin, green leafy vegetables, selected nuts and seeds.

The aromatherapy treatment mainly involved skin and anti-stress essential oils such as bergamot, lavender and juniper. Chamomile was also introduced later in the program. Juniper is a good detoxifier and this was chosen because of the caffeine in her diet. It should be noted that the withdrawal symptoms of caffeine include nausea and headaches.

Helen received a full-body aromatherapy massage with gentle movements over the affected areas using these oils once a fortnight. She was also encouraged to use half a cap of this aromatherapy blend in her bath.

Two weeks after the first treatment Helen's skin had cleared dramatically, with only a small patch of psoriasis remaining on her neck and back. She had experienced a mild headache for two days early in the treatment, which was put down to the detoxifying process. She reported feeling more relaxed and less bothered by negative emotions.

> Helen was massaged again with the same blend of oils. On her next visit the psoriasis had improved once more. It had flared at one stage after an argument, but was helped by inhaling the oils.
>
> I made Helen a nourishing base cream, with added evening primrose oil, a vitamin E capsule (scar healing), lavender, bergamot and chamomile, to use on her skin.
>
> With additional stress-management advice, Helen's psoriasis is very much under control.

Weight gain

Research from the University of Sydney shows that girls automatically gain weight when they reach puberty and begin menstruating. The body mass of non-menstruating girls (aged between 11 and 15 years) was compared with that of menstruating teenagers of the same age. The menstruating group had a larger body mass.

Aroma aid: While nothing can replace a balanced, low-fat diet and regular exercise, aromatherapy can assist in weight management. A blend of lemon, geranium and cypress will help to relieve congestion and remove excess fluid.

Place 12 drops of cypress, 8 of lemon and 7 of geranium in 50ml (1⅔ fl oz) of apricot kernel oil. Massage the body after your morning shower with a small amount of the mixture in your cupped hand. Concentrate on the 'podgy' areas. This is a great anti-cellulite blend.

LOOKING GOOD

STRONG NAILS

When I was a teenager, the quality of your nails and hair was a benchmark as to whether you were 'in' or not. Bitten, flaky nails just didn't make the grade. Here is a great nail-strengthening aromatherapy treat for your nails.

Add warm water to two small bowls (enough to cover your nails), then add 5 drops of lemon essential oil to each. Soak your nails for 3–5 minutes, remove them and wipe dry. Repeat this 2 or 3 times each week until the desired strength is reached.

The mineral silica, which is found in tablet form in health food stores, is also excellent for strong nails.

Shiny Hair

The hair is our crowning glory. The shinier it is, the healthier it looks.

If you have dark hair, add 6 drops of sandalwood to 500ml (16 fl oz) of warm water. Rinse through the hair after washing and conditioning (avoid the eye area).

To add highlights to blonde or light brown hair, chamomile is the answer. Boil 750ml (24 fl oz) of water and place 3 chamomile teabags in it. Let the mixture stand for 5 minutes. Remove the teabags and add 3 drops of chamomile essential oil to the mixture. Rinse through the hair after washing and conditioning.

Healthy Skin

See Chapter 8 for easy instructions on how to identify the essential oils that suit your skin type and how to make your own natural beauty products. I seem to get inspired on Sunday afternoons to pamper myself and make my aromatherapy wardrobe for the week.

1. Cleanse morning and night with a natural cleanser that has 2 drops of your skin type's essential oil in it. Place a small amount onto cottonwool pads and gently wipe over the face, avoiding the eye area. One cottonwool pad can be easily split in half, saving you money.
2. Make your own aromatherapy toner; it's easy! Place the suitable toner onto cottonwool pads and again wipe over the same area.

3. Select the essential oils for your skin type and place them in a nourishing base oil or cream. Gently massage it into the face.

Remember to drink lots of water, eat a balanced diet and take regular exercise.

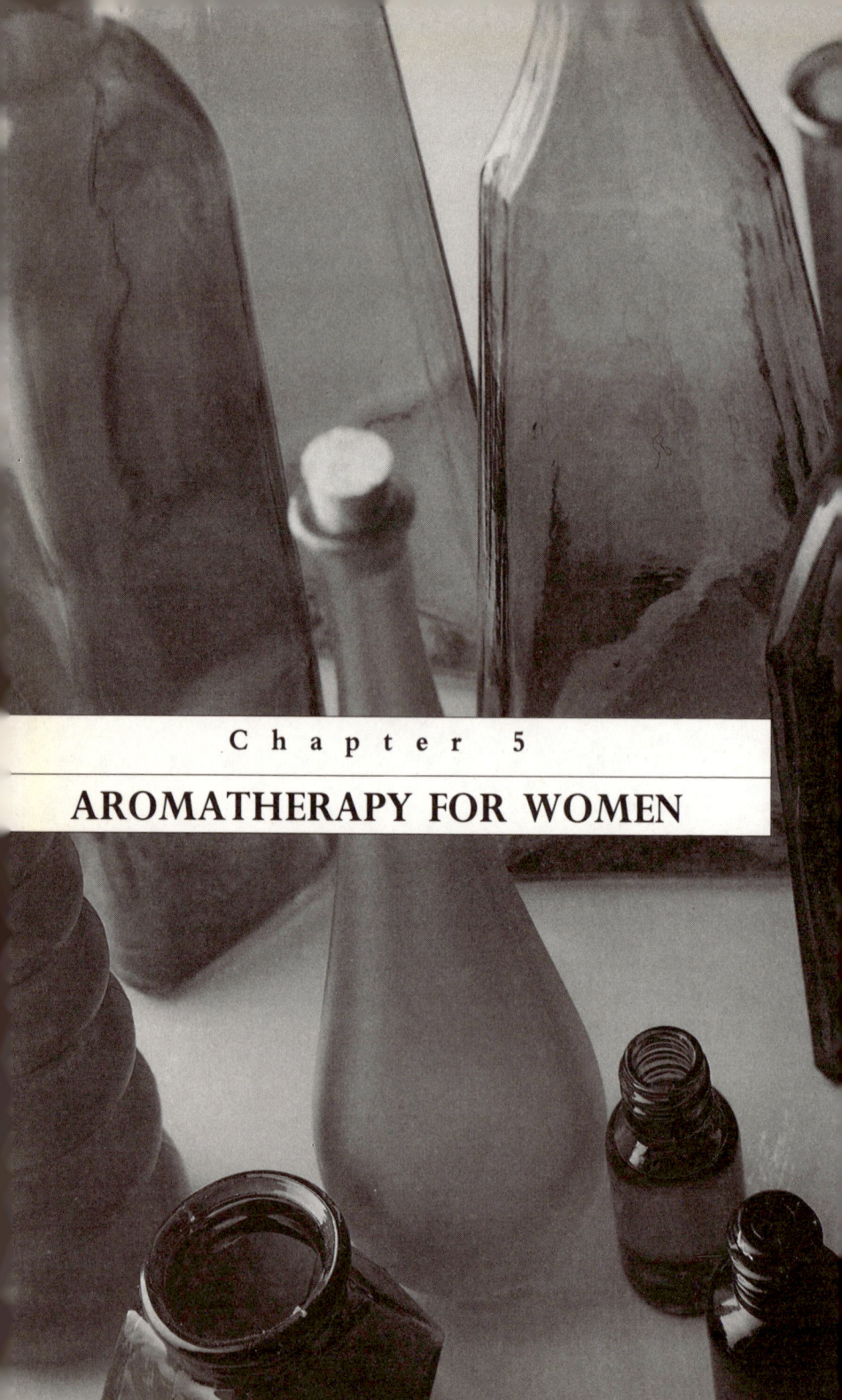

Chapter 5
AROMATHERAPY FOR WOMEN

The enticing world of aromatherapy can touch a woman's life in so many different ways. Whether you're in your 20s or 60s, calming, uplifting, energising and therapeutic essential oils can help you to enjoy life more.

It's just as well that help is at hand because women statistically appear to be busier than ever. The figures for higher education in recent years state that 53.5 per cent of enrolments are female. In 1995, women made up 42 per cent of the workforce, compared with 25 per cent in 1961. Fifty per cent of sole parents (90 per cent of which are women) are in the workforce. And one study showed that 42 per cent of female senior executives also did most of the housework, compared with 4 per cent of executive males. Sounds exhausting, doesn't it? So, we're studying and working more and, in the case of some working women and mothers, maintaining the home. Whether you're at home, at work or both, aromatherapy has much to offer you.

AROMATHERAPY AND WOMEN

Dinner Parties

The casual approach to dinner with close friends does not send the blood pressure rising as much as those 'have tos' involving business associates or distant relatives passing by.

If you're wanting to avoid awkward silences during dinner, place 2 drops of neroli and 6 of orange in an aromatherapy burner. Light the burner's candle around an hour before your guests arrive and remember to top it up with water and essential oils during the night. Sit back and watch the laughter and conversations rise.

Hangover

See Chapter 6

Home Sweet Home

Aromatherapy makes sense for different rooms: 'clean' smells for the bathroom, welcoming odours for the entrance and alluring scents for the boudoir. Use the essential oils in a potpourri, on a herb pillow or in an aromatherapy burner.
Entrance: orange, lavender, geranium, lemon
Lounge room: lavender, bergamot, clary sage, cedarwood
Bathroom: lemon, pine, eucalyptus, tea-tree, peppermint, rosemary
Bedroom: sandalwood, rose, patchouli, ylang-ylang

Housework Blues

Cleaning up your own mess is usually easier than cleaning up someone else's. To help you get through this sometimes mundane task, try this energising blend: place 4 drops of lemon and rosemary in an aromatherapy burner. This will get you up and moving.

'I'm Positive'

No matter what the facade, no one is positive 100 per cent of the time. Life and emotions come in cycles. However, there are many things you can do, such as exercise, eating well, positive self-talk and relaxation, to help you maintain a lighter frame of mind. The citrus oils (bergamot, orange, lemon, neroli, petitgrain) are the most uplifting of all essential oils. Take regular sniffs from a vaporiser or tissue.

Romance

Imagine the warm glow of an aromatherapy burner subtly reflecting off your partner's oiled body and sensual aromas filling the room. Soft music plays quietly in the background (set the CD on repeat) and a lovingly decanted massage oil sits near the bed. A romantic atmosphere for you and your partner is guaranteed.

This alluring atmosphere can be achieved by using the essential oils of rose, ylang-ylang and patchouli. Place 2 drops★ of each oil in a burner or in 20ml (⅔ fl oz) of sweet almond oil for an erotic massage blend. A drop of diluted rose on your pulse points and on dark-coloured lingerie is highly recommended.

★These essential oils are all base notes (see Chapter 9), so I have reduced the total number of drops in the burner and massage oil.

STUDY

See Chapter 4

TIME OUT

This is a necessary part of healthy living. Those who don't take time for themselves often end up snappy and stressed. Unwinding and letting go of anxiety, worry, stress and tension not only helps you to feel better but often clarifies your thoughts and situation.

Frankincense is a fortifying and comforting essential oil, and mixed with the nerve tonics bergamot and lavender will give you the relaxation you need. Use the oils in your favourite aromatherapy way: in a bath, massage blend, burner, or potpourri, or on a tissue. As a guide, in a burner use 2 drops of frankincense and 3 drops each of bergamot and lavender.

Aromatherapy and meditation exercise

Meditation increases your energy and vitality, and helps you to let go of anxieties. Twenty minutes of meditation daily can have a very positive influence on your life. You will feel more centred and able to face almost anything. There are various forms of meditation, but one of my favourites combines visualisation and aromatherapy.

1. In a quiet room sit comfortably on the floor or in a chair. Add 5 drops of myrrh and 3 drops of frankincense

to an aromatherapy burner, and place it nearby. These oils will allow deep relaxation and support you through the meditation.

2. With your eyes closed, start to take three slow, deep breaths and feel your muscles letting go and relaxing. Become aware of the aromas wafting up from the vaporiser; inhale them and let their relaxing properties meander through every part of your body.
3. Now pick a colour (pastels, white or golden light are my favourites) that makes you feel good. Imagine you are breathing in your chosen colour and feel the pleasant sensation of that colour expanding through your body. See it extending outwards more and more, positively affecting the people around you.
4. Next visualise yourself walking along a beautiful path (if you find visualising difficult, just imagine you are there). You could be walking along a beach, a forest floor, a moon beam, whatever feels right for you. Up ahead you see a clearing. Head for the beautiful area that you have created.
5. Sit down and visualise yourself with your aromatherapy burner beside you in this beautiful place. Slowly inhale the frankincense and myrrh several times. You can instantaneously feel their benefits. You feel completely relaxed. Become aware of how good it feels to be totally relaxed. Remember the feeling. Sit with it for a time.
6. When you're ready, get up and walk back to your beautiful path. Back to the present. Begin to wiggle your hands and feet and feel the energy returning to them. Open your eyes and have a good stretch.

When you are faced with anxiety or stress, step back, take three deep breaths and consciously remember how good you felt when you were relaxed. See yourself relaxed and calm (just like you were while visualising) ... and you will be.

Friendly massage

Practise the foot, shoulder and head massage mentioned in Chapter 3. When visiting a friend, pick a rose from the garden, take your essential oil kit and footbath with you. A relaxing foot massage using essential oils and rose petal-soaked water doesn't take long, and you might as well throw in a pedicure! My friends adore my visits. (See Chapter 6 for an easy back massage.)

TRAVEL

See Chapter 6

WEDDING DAY

You're exuberant, you're excited ... and possibly a little anxious. Flowers? Hair? Make-up? Dress? Catering? Family? Guests? And so on. To calm you down so that you can fully take in this special day, here's a blend for you.

Put 3 drops of geranium and 2 of sandalwood onto a tissue. Take three deep breaths from the tissue every 30 minutes until you feel balanced and centred.

MOTHERHOOD

Some mothers say that the only time they get to rest is when their children are in bed. A bath of geranium and orange (3 drops each) and sandalwood (2 drops) can help a mum to rebalance and restore her nervous system at the end of a long day.

If you are feeling worn out and fatigued, add rosemary (2 drops) with lemon and peppermint (3 drops each) to an aromatherapy burner. If you feel your anger and impatience getting out of hand, instead of chastising the child, sniff a few drops of rose, chamomile or cypress from a tissue.

Mums handle crises in different ways. Some are cool and calm (until later) and others panic straight away. Neroli is the key essential oil for shock; sniff it from a tissue as soon as possible, or place a few drops in a base oil and rub it into your wrist pulse points.

Work

The first time you put an aromatherapy burner on your work desk, you may get a few funny looks . . . but persevere. After a few minutes of inhaling the potent vapour, even cynical workmates will be feeling less stressed and clearer in the mind.

Use 8 drops in total from any three essential oils from these groups: the anti-stress essential oils — orange, bergamot, lavender, geranium, frankincense or sandalwood; or the energising, memory boosters — rosemary, basil, lemongrass or lemon.

Make Your Own Perfume

Make your own perfumed masterpiece. You can design an aromatherapy perfume that will envelop you in pleasure, and you will also know exactly what has gone into it (not synthetic copies of natural odours as with many commercially available perfumes). Experiment with a small quantity first until you have a blend you love. My favourites are jasmine, mandarin and sandalwood.

Mix 10 drops of your essential oil blend with 15–20mls of base oil (depending on how strong you want the perfume) and pour it into an elegant glass bottle.

Place 1–2 drops onto your pulse points. Renew the perfume halfway through the day.

Relationship Endings

Separation, finishing a relationship, divorce and death are all situations that cause pain and grief. Besides talking to someone you trust or seeing a professional counsellor (if appropriate), you can use essential oils to help you deal with the emotions surrounding these circumstances and to help you move forward in life.

Bergamot, neroli and rose can be placed in an aromatherapy burner, used in the bath (for bath and burner, use 4 drops of bergamot and 2 drops of each rose and neroli — the 2–2.5 per cent dilutions) or inhaled from a tissue (use a few drops of one oil or 1 drop of each three).

AROMATHERAPY AND AILMENTS IN WOMEN

Cellulite
See Chapter 4

Cystitis
See Chapter 4

Digestive disorders
Bloating, flatulence and constipation (see Chapter 4), diarrhoea (see Chapter 3). Heartburn will be covered in the 'Pregnancy' section of this chapter.

Fatal illness
Cancer, AIDS, advanced heart disease, for instance. People often experience emotional symptoms such as depression, grief, anger, fear and shock when they discover they have a serious or potentially fatal illness. Professional guidance is often necessary at this time.
Aroma aid: Inhaling a few drops of the following essential oils from a tissue or using them in the sponge bath or compress can

be helpful: rose or neroli for grief or shock, chamomile or clary sage for fear, ylang-ylang or rose for anger, and bergamot, orange, lavender and clary sage to lift the spirits. These essential oils can also be of benefit to the carer.

Aromatherapists, with the medical practitioner's consent, may also support the physical well-being of the immune, nervous or indicated system of the person. They may also work with centres such as The Quest for Life Foundation, supporting people facing life-threatening illnesses.

Frigidity

A lack of sexual desire. Frigidity can be present for many reasons, among them hormonal imbalance and a history of sexual abuse. Counselling is vital for the latter cause. Essential oils can also help this situation.

Aroma aid: Regular massages and baths with a combination of three oils (2 drops of each in a bath, or with 20ml (⅔ fl oz) of a base oil for massage), choosing from neroli, patchouli, rose, sandalwood and ylang-ylang.

Haemorrhoids

The blood-filled 'cushions' that are contained in the wall of the anus become enlarged. There are three main degrees of haemorrhoids, the first being bleeding and minor pain because of fissures (cracks) in the anus, with the symptoms progressively advancing to the third degree where the haemorrhoids protrude and need to be forced back inside the anus.

Aroma aid: To ease the pain caused by fissures, take a daily hipbath with equal drops (4) of cypress and juniper. For advanced haemorrhoids, a swab using cypress and juniper would also be beneficial.

Other: A balanced high-fibre diet containing wholefoods can assist in alleviating symptoms. Avoid white bread, highly processed foods and large quantities of red meat in the diet. Witch-hazel is the herb of choice for this condition, along with bioflavonoids and vitamin E.

Headache

Pain that is felt superficially or deep within the skull. Headaches can be brought on by emotional stress, fatigue, allergies or structural disorders.

HEADACHE: JULIE'S STORY

Julie's painful, throbbing (and uncharacteristic) headache began while she was sitting at her work desk. It progressively got worse and she gave me a call before returning home.

Her case history did not consist of allergies, fatigue or a physical cause such as a fall. There was, however, a stressful situation with her boss, which we spoke about and has since been resolved. I called Julie later that evening and she was symptom-free. If her headaches had persisted I would have referred her on for the necessary tests.

Treatment

I told her to place neat lavender on her temples and at the back of her neck where the main source of pain was located. When I saw Julie that afternoon her pain had eased. As she said, 'It didn't cure it, but it decreased the intensity of the pain.' I proceeded to massage her scalp, neck and shoulders with a lavender massage blend. And I asked Julie to hold the acupressure point for headache relief, which is located between the thumb and index finger, during the treatment.

I also recommended two 65mg magnesium phosphate tablets to be taken initially and again (if required) in another two hours' time. Magnesium is the neuromuscular mineral that relaxes tense muscles. In my experience, these tablets are just as effective as allopathic headache tablets for stress headaches.

Aroma aid: Apply a few drops of neat lavender to the temple or forehead area. Add 5 drops of lavender to 10ml of sweet almond oil and ask a person nearby to gently massage your shoulder, scalp and neck area.

Herpes
See Chapter 4

High blood pressure
See Chapter 6

Leucorrhoea
An abnormally large discharge of whitish or yellowish mucus from the vaginal opening, usually due to infection of the lower reproductive area by *Trichomonas vaginalis*, for example.
Aroma aid: Douche with 6 drops of tea-tree oil in half a litre of warm water. This can be done once or twice daily until symptoms reduce. Allergies can inadvertently cause the symptoms experienced above. If they consume too much dairy or sugar, some women comment on the manifestation of the thick white discharge.

Low blood pressure
A decline in arterial pressure below the 'normal' range (120/80).
Aroma aid: Place 3 drops of lemon and rosemary and 2 drops of thyme in an aromatherapy burner. Make a massage blend using the above oils (with appropriate doses) into 20–40ml (⅔–1⅓ fl oz) of base oil, and massage once per week.

Menopause
A time in a woman's life (usually between 45 and 55 years) when she stops ovulating and menstruating. Periods may stop suddenly or gradually decrease. The change in the balance of sex hormones in the body, which occurs at this time, can lead to hot flushes, palpitations, moodiness and dryness of the vaginal mucous membrane.

Aroma aid: Regular massage with rose, geranium and cypress can help to alleviate the symptoms of menopause by balancing the hormonal roller-coaster effect. To 50ml (1⅔ fl oz) of sweet almond oil add 4 drops of rose, 9 drops of geranium and 12 of cypress. Use 5ml of this massage oil in a bath. To use in an aromatherapy burner, add 1 drop of rose, 3 drops of geranium and 4 drops of cypress.

Menopause: Debbie's Story

Debbie, aged 53, was experiencing daily flushes, a decrease in her sex drive (which was causing problems in her relationship) and a marked lack of self-confidence. The flushing in particular was 'embarrassing' and hard to cope with. For this reason she dreaded going out of the house. Debbie was in a low-risk category of osteoporosis (there was no incidence in her family and she was heavy set). She wanted to avoid hormone replacement therapy and came to me for a natural alternative.

Treatment

Using the menopause blend above, I massaged Debbie once weekly for three weeks and gave her the blend to wear as a 'perfume', to use in the bath and in a room vaporiser. Over a three-week period her symptoms greatly improved. She really seemed like a new woman sitting across from me. Her confidence had increased, there were no more flushes and her libido had returned to normal.

I recommended that she continue using the aromatherapy blend in her bath and vaporiser.

Premenstrual syndrome
See Chapter 4

Thrush
A yeast infection caused by *Candida albicans* that mainly affects the tongue, inside cheeks, vagina and skin. A white 'cottage cheese'-like discharge is a noted symptom.
Aroma aid: Tea-tree oil pessaries are available commercially for insertion into the vagina. A regular douche using 6 drops of tea-tree oil is also beneficial.
Other: The diet plays a big role in the management of this condition. Avoiding sugar, alcohol, yeast-containing products and mushrooms among other foods is vital. Your naturopath can help with a detailed diet menu. *Lactobacillus acidophilus* is a favourable flora that can combat thrush. The capsules or powder are recommended. The antifungal properties of garlic are also effective in combating this irritating disorder.

Vaginal irritation
Itching or discomfort in the vaginal area after sexual intercourse using a condom.
Aroma aid: Add 6 drops of tea-tree oil in a litre of warm water and use as a douche to alleviate the symptoms.

Varicose veins
The superficial veins of the legs are usually affected by varicosities — distended, tortuous veins. Nature's ingredients that have astringent properties and improve the blood supply to the veins are indicated here.
Aroma aid: Make a warm compress using rosemary (2 drops), cypress (3 drops) and lemon (3 drops). Apply regularly to the varicosed area.

Weight gain
See Chapter 4

> ## Cleopatra's Bath Secrets
>
> Have you ever wondered about the secrets of Cleopatra's long-lasting beauty? Some say it was her daily bathing rituals, which incorporated the exotic and youth-sustaining essential oils.
>
> Mix 1 tablespoon of full-cream milk powder with a little water to form a loose paste. Add to this 2 drops of the rejuvenating essential oils of neroli, rose and lavender. Stir and pour the mixture into the bath while the water is running.
>
> While you are in the bath, take the time to pamper yourself. Apply a clay and fruit facial masque to suit your skin type (see Chapter 8), or persuade your 'Mark Antony' to wash and massage your back.

PREGNANCY, CHILDBIRTH AND POST-BIRTH

At this special time in your life it's natural that you will want to take good care of your health. This includes eating a balanced diet, exercising, avoiding stimulants such as coffee, cigarettes and alcohol and keeping a positive mental attitude.

It has also been proven that taking a good multivitamin and folic acid supplement daily prior to conception and in the early months of pregnancy can reduce the risk of having a baby with spina bifida or a low birth weight.

Aromatherapy can enhance this important time in your life by helping you to conquer the common symptoms during pregnancy (morning sickness and heartburn) and to reduce the pain and discomfort of labour. After the birth, if mastitis, sore nipples, poor lactation or depression is a problem, aromatherapy has a few gentle ideas to help.

Aromatherapy during Pregnancy

Essential oil blends when formulated by a qualified practitioner can only benefit a mum-to-be. The following oils are used in treatments after the first trimester (three months) of pregnancy: lavender, frankincense, sandalwood, mandarin, tangerine, geranium, lemongrass, cypress and ylang-ylang. They should be used at half the adult dose; that is, for a massage, instead of using 1 drop every 2ml of base oil, use 1 drop every 4ml of base oil.

There are a few essential oils that are *not* recommended during pregnancy because of their abortive or neurotoxic properties. These oils are mentioned in Chapter 9 but will be repeated here for convenience. If in doubt, don't use an essential oil even in a vaporiser. Ask your aromatherapist for advice.

Avoid during Pregnancy

The pregnancy avoidance list refers to the 30 essential oils mentioned in Chapter 9, they include:
basil, cedarwood, clary sage★, fennel, juniper, peppermint, marjoram, myrrh, rosemary, sage, thyme.
★Can be used during labour

Constipation
This uncomfortable condition occurs during pregnancy because of the increasing pressure placed on the intestines. A high-fibre, wholefood diet and plenty of water are required at this time.
Aroma aid: Place 10 drops of orange in 40ml (1⅓ fl oz) of apricot kernel or sweet almond oil, then massage it over the abdomen regularly. You can also place 5ml of this oil in a bath.

Heartburn

As the baby grows, it places more pressure on the stomach area and acid escapes from the stomach, resulting in a rising burning sensation. You can do more than just prop yourself up with pillows.
Aroma aid: Inhale 1 drop of sandalwood and 1 drop of mandarin from a tissue.

Morning sickness

This inconvenient condition usually occurs during the first three months of pregnancy. Having said that, I do know of several women who have suffered morning sickness through most of the pregnancy!
Aroma aid: A lavender (4 drops) compress on the abdomen is recommended. The powdered root of ginger (available in tablet form) has also been found to be safe and effective against morning sickness.

AROMATHERAPY PREGNANCY MASSAGE

A pregnant woman feels pampered and soothed after experiencing a deluxe massage at the skilled hands of an aromatherapist. The enchanting atmosphere of flowers, aromatic vapours, relaxing music and soft lighting in a warm room can do nothing but relax. During pregnancy, a massage once every month and more often towards birth is recommended. There is a special massage technique used by aromatherapists during pregnancy, as it would obviously be unwise to lay a big, round tummy 'face down' onto a massage table.

1. After selecting the essential oils and natural beauty products for the massage and facial, the mum-to-be sits on the table with her legs to one side. She leaves her underpants on and has a towel around her front area. Over the towel is a large pillow, which she

holds with both arms. Her feet are supported by a bench.

The aromatherapist works from behind, using the unique aromatherapy massage techniques to gently massage the whole back area, shoulders, neck and scalp. The full support of the pillow, table and bench allows the woman to relax totally and enjoy the experience. If a cotton blanket is placed over her back and shoulders, the woman is in an ideal position for a soothing lavender footbath.

Some practitioners lay the pregnant woman on her right side and fully support her abdomen, head, neck and knees with pillows. They then work on the back area in this position.

2. When it's time to move to the front of the body, the table is prepared with strategically placed pillows and towels for support — two or more large pillows under the upper back and head, two under the knees and legs. The pillows are moved until the pregnant woman feels comfortable. The towel remains on the front and she is covered with a cotton blanket.

An aromatherapist will usually work from the head down, starting with a scalp massage, moving on to a full facial (a masque can be applied at this time), including massaging the neck, chest and shoulder area. Next the therapist works on the arms and hands and the abdomen area. Pregnant women often report a soothing benefit from having their tummies rubbed during massage. Then down to the legs and feet. If a masque has been applied, it is now removed and an aromatherapy moisturiser is applied to the face.

Stretch marks
As the breasts and abdomen grow, so do tiny scars in the underlying skin layers.
Aroma aid: Massage the chest and abdomen morning and night with the following formula: to 45ml (1½ fl oz) of apricot kernel oil with 5ml of wheatgerm oil (it contains scar-healing vitamin E), add 7 drops of lavender, 5 drops of tangerine and 2 drops of frankincense. This is a very effective blend when used regularly. A course of a zinc supplement can also help to reduce scarring.

AROMATHERAPY DURING LABOUR

Maternity sections of hospitals are becoming more aware of the benefits of aromatherapy in their wards. Some hospitals have an in-house aromatherapist, who massages and assists women about to give birth. My, how times have changed.

Room sterilisation
Hospitals have that characteristic unpleasant 'sterile' smell. To improve the odour and to provide your own antiseptic for your room, try the following.
Aroma aid: Place 4 drops of lavender, 2 drops of tea-tree and 2 drops of lemon into an aromatherapy burner. Top up as required.

Pain relief
Most women say that the pain experienced during labour and childbirth is indescribable. Aromatherapy can help to ease the pain. Have a loving partner standing by to look after you.
Aroma aid: Massaging the lower back with firm rhythmic pressure can be helpful during the first few hours of labour. Use 6 drops of clary sage, 4 drops of ylang-ylang and 2 drops of neroli in 50ml (1⅔ fl oz) of sweet almond or apricot kernel oil. This will ease the pain and reduce the emotional stress, too.

A clary sage compress using 4–8 drops of the essential oil

can often work instantly for pain relief. The homoeopathic remedy Arnica can also decrease the pain and increase the healing time of the reproductive tissues. Mum and Dad will benefit from a practical session with an aromatherapist. A personalised 'Childbirth' kit can be made for you.

Aromatherapy after the Birth

Postnatal care is just as important as antenatal care. Mothers can easily get exhausted by the extra demands placed on their body and time. Once again, aromatherapy can make this time a pleasant one. It is vital that a baby never suck on an essential oil treated area. Always wash the nipple/breast before feeding.

Lactation difficulties

Sometimes a mother can have difficulty producing sufficient milk for a child. The desire is there, but the milk just isn't flowing. Or, they experience the opposite problem of an excess of milk.

Aroma aid: Fennel is excellent for inducing a good milk supply. Drink fennel tea (available from health food stores) and massage the breasts twice daily with 2 drops of fennel in 10ml of sweet almond or apricot kernel oil, until normal milk supply has resumed. Sage tea is recommended for reducing the milk supply.

Mastitis

This painful condition can manifest when the milk duct in a nipple is damaged or clogged. Inflammation of the mammary glands can occur if the breast is not completely emptied of milk.

Aroma aid: Apply a cold compress using chamomile (1 drop), lavender (2 drops) and rose (1 drop) to the area regularly. Common cabbage leaves also do a terrific healing job.

Sore nipples

All that sucking and pressure on the tender nipples can cause cracks and bleeding in the area.
Aroma aid: Gently apply 1 drop of rose and lavender in 20ml (⅔ fl oz) of sweet almond or apricot kernel oil to the nipple between feeds.

Postnatal depression

Having a baby can be overwhelming. Suddenly there are extra responsibilities and demands on your time. Some mums can experience depression. Catch yourself and treat it early. Seek professional help if symptoms persist.
Aroma aid: A blend of antidepressant essential oils such as mandarin, lavender and sandalwood can change this situation around quickly. Use 4 drops each of mandarin and lavender and 2 of sandalwood in an aromatherapy burner. And place a few drops of each onto a tissue and inhale regularly.

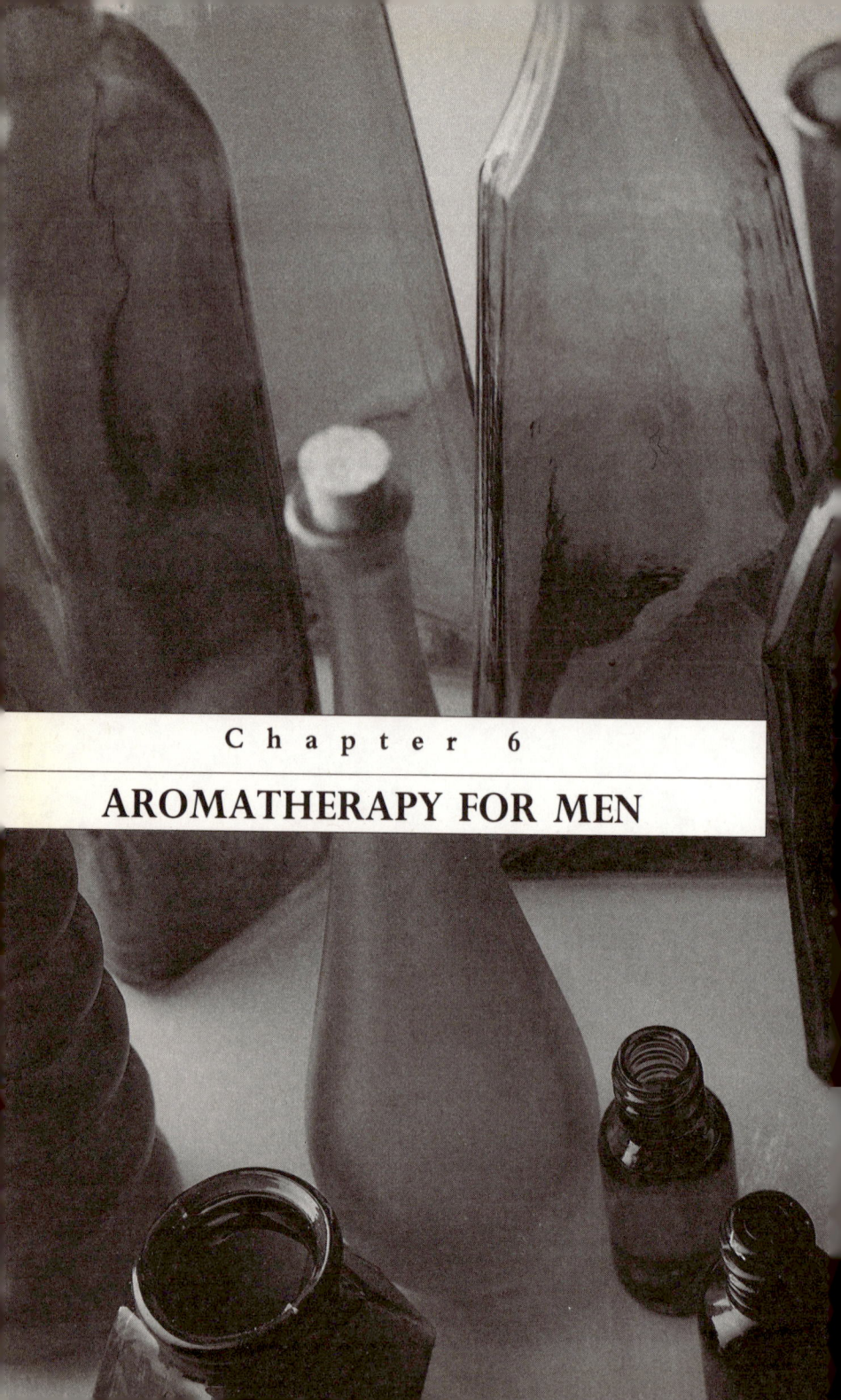

Chapter 6

AROMATHERAPY FOR MEN

Modern men may not wish to place aromatic wax cones on their heads as the Pharaohs did, but there is no doubt that aromatherapy is becoming as popular among men as it is with women.

In fact, the use of essential oils was very much a male-dominated pastime in ancient times. The scent shops of Rome, for instance, were used much as our coffee shops and bars are today — as places in which to meet and exchange opinions.

Even the famous first-century emperor Nero extravagantly indulged in the use of essential oils. Not only was his body scented, but the walls and floors of his buildings were aromatic. The dining-room walls had movable square tiles that, when turned, allowed flowers and essential oils to fall into the room.

AROMATHERAPY AND MEN

Jump in My Car

Some people spend long hours in their car each day, so wouldn't it be great if there was something that helped to decrease the stress of dealing with traffic?

Place a few drops of cedarwood, sandalwood or orange onto a cottonwool ball and put it in a handy spot in the car. The anti-stress aromas will waft past your nostrils, calming any anxiety before it stirs. You might even enjoy the journey.

Travel

Being on the road or in the air can easily cause fatigue. But there's that crucial meeting to attend or that client to meet, so you have to be alert!

An aromatherapy peppermint mist spray can do wonders to refresh a tired face or mind. If you are taking long trips where you aren't driving, try inhaling from a tissue 1 drop of vetiver and 2 each of marjoram and lavender to help you sleep.

Hangover

We'll all probably experience a hangover at least once in our lives. For some, it's a regular event. Prevention is always better than cure, as they say, but if it's too late for that ... Placing a few drops of peppermint onto a tissue and inhaling regularly is a solution for the nausea. A cold compress using 5 drops of lavender and 3 of geranium placed onto the forehead or nape of the neck can do wonders to relieve the inevitable headache.

Holidays

Before setting off, take a little time to pack the following holiday first-aid kit.

Holiday First-aid Kit

Contents: Lavender, peppermint, tea-tree, cotton gauze cloth, cottonwool, small quantity of base oil.

Lavender

This versatile essential oil that can be used to treat headaches, mild burns and insect bites among other ailments. Remember, lavender is the only essential oil that can be applied directly onto the skin.

Headaches: Massage a few drops of lavender onto the temples. Or make a compress with 8 drops of lavender in a bowl of water. Apply the pre-soaked gauze cloth to the neck or painful area.

Mild burns: After a cold compress has been applied for

5–10 minutes, gently place neat lavender onto the burn. Repeat again after 3–4 hours.
Insect bites: Lavender is a natural insect repellent. It can also help to ease the 'bite' from an insect when applied neat.

Peppermint

This can relieve indigestion, heartburn, general tummy upsets and catarrh.
Indigestion and heartburn: Massage a blend of 2 drops of peppermint and a teaspoon of base oil onto the stomach and abdomen area.
Catarrh or sinusitis: Place a few drops of peppermint and tea-tree oil in a bowl of hot water and, using the old towel over the head trick, inhale the vapours to help unblock the nasal passages and clear catarrh.

Tea-tree

This oil is well known for its potent antiseptic properties. It can be useful in the treatment of abrasions.
Abrasions: Wash the wound with a preparation of 8 drops of tea-tree oil in half a cup of warm, pre-boiled water. Leave uncovered (if possible). If an adhesive dressing is required, put 1 drop of the oil onto the gauzed area before applying.

HOUSEWORK BLUES

See Chapter 5

WORKING, WORKING, WORKING

For those of you who are climbing the corporate ladder or building your own business, there just aren't enough hours in the day. While this situation is fine in the short term, 15-hour (plus) working days are not conducive to a balanced life or relationship in the long haul.

The concentration aromatherapy blend of rosemary, basil and lemon can help to improve your efficiency so that you achieve more in a shorter space of time. Bergamot (4 drops), cedarwood (1 drop) and lavender (3 drops) in an office aromatherapy burner or bath at the end of the day will help you to stay calm and will ease stress.

Romance

When you give your partner some roses, place a few drops of the aphrodisiac essential oils rose, ylang-ylang, sandalwood or patchouli onto the back of the card or even on the bud of the flower. Or purchase (or make) a 'romance' essential oil kit and send it with an aromatherapy burner to someone you want to get close to. It's only a subtle hint!

Massaging a partner can be a very stimulating part of foreplay. Add to this the aphrodisiac essential oils and hold the phone calls ...

Popping the Question

It's a clear-cut decision for some; for others it's a 'Will I or won't I?' event. If in doubt, don't. Some people know what they want, but they just need a little confidence and courage to state their intentions of marriage. Aromatherapy can help to calm the nerves and boost your confidence.

Place 1 drop of vetiver and 2 drops of frankincense into 6ml of a base oil and rub the mixture into your solar plexus (just between the lower ribs).

Wedding Day

You're feeling great (well, that depends if your bucks party was the night before), but you're also feeling a little nervous. What can you do?

The aromatherapy solution in 'Popping the Question' will also serve you well here. It will calm and give confidence to allow you to enjoy fully your special day.

Fatherhood

Having children or babies in your life can be fun and at other times frustrating and exhausting. Children can't seem to be angels all of the time. Whether you're a 'home-dad' or a 'working-dad', aromatherapy essential oils can help you.

If impatience is a problem, place a few drops of bergamot or cypress onto a tissue and inhale; for frustration or anger, add ylang-ylang; and for fatigue, add lemongrass or rosemary.

Handyman

Working with your hands — sawing, hammering, gardening, concreting or just fixing the things that need to be fixed — can give you calluses and aches in your muscles and bones.

For a healing blend, add lavender (3 drops), tea-tree (2 drops) in 10g of vitamin E cream (available from pharmacies and health food stores) to your hands regularly. After a hard day's work, add 5 drops of lavender and 3 of rosemary to a bath to alleviate your aches and pains.

Relationship Endings

Separating, finishing a relationship, divorce and even death are all situations that cause pain and grief. Besides talking to someone you trust and counselling (if appropriate), essential oils can help you to deal with the emotions surrounding these circumstances and help you to move forward in life.

The essential oils bergamot, marjoram and neroli can be

placed in an aromatherapy burner, used in the bath (for bath and burner, use 4 drops of bergamot, 3 drops of marjoram and 1 drop of neroli) or inhaled from a tissue (use a few drops of one oil or 1 drop of each three).

AROMATHERAPY AND COMMON MALE AILMENTS

There are a few health conditions that may come with being male — prostate disorders, impotence and the male menopause, for instance. And there are others that have a higher incidence in males.

Arthritis

Inflammation of one or more joints, characterised by pain, redness and swelling. Rheumatoid arthritis and osteoarthritis are the two most common forms that occur in men.

Aroma aid: Rosemary, juniper and lavender can be made into a lotion and rubbed gently onto the joints. Add 11 drops of lavender, 8 of juniper and 6 of rosemary to 50ml (1⅔ fl oz) of apricot kernel oil. Apply this to the affected joints twice daily.

Other: Fish oil capsules and celery seed tablets or fluid extract are beneficial in relieving the symptoms of arthritis.

ARTHRITIS: JOHN'S STORY

John, aged 63, came to me after suffering from osteoarthritis for 20 years. The pain and stiffness in his joints had been worse since a car accident six years ago, and seemed to be increasing, particularly in his right hand and lower back. John lives in a cold climate and likes to play a weekly game of golf. He came to see me because he was feeling depressed about his lack of mobility.

Treatment

On the first visit I massaged John, paying attention to his lower back and hand, with pepper, rosemary and eucalyptus to warm and improve circulation with the antirheumatic and antidepressant essential oil, lavender.

After the massage he reported feeling calmer and less stiff. I gave John a bottle of the blend and instructed him to use a teaspoonful in the bath. The next week John said that he had still experienced a little pain and stiffness during the week, but that he felt more mobile. I repeated this blend in a massage.

A telephone conversation with John during the next week confirmed that his mobility and pain had markedly decreased. Then a setback — he tripped over a garden hose and injured his lower back. His osteopath gave him three treatments. After a week's absence he returned, and I continued weekly aromatherapy massage for the next four weeks. After the accident I substituted clary sage for rosemary to lift his spirits.

John is now almost pain-free and his mobility has increased, allowing him to enjoy his game of golf. He books in for a massage once a month to ensure his old achey problems don't return.

Athlete's foot

The common name for tinea pedis, a fungal infection that affects more men than women. Tinea appears as a reddish inflamed surface between the toes, which sloughs off leaving a raw area beneath.

Aroma aid: Tea-tree, myrrh and thyme (in combination) are very potent antifungal essential oils. Add 2 drops of each oil into 1 cup of cornflour. Wash and dry the feet before applying the blend. The toes can be dusted with the mixture twice daily. Keep the feet dry and out of enclosed shoes as much as possible.

Tinea: Tea-tree Oil Study

A study carried out in 1992 shows the effects of tea-tree oil in the treatment of tinea pedis.

Method

One hundred and four people completed the randomised, double-blind trial, which evaluated the efficacy of 10 per cent w/w tea-tree oil cream with 1 per cent tolnaftate (a common drug for tinea) and a Sorbolene placebo cream.

Results

All three groups showed improvements in their condition (reduced scaling, inflammation, itching and burning) — 24 out of the 37 in the tea-tree oil group, 19 out of 33 in the tolnaftate group and 14 out of 34 for the placebo group — after the month-long treatment. The placebo group's improvement was thought to have occurred because of the basic hygiene procedures of washing and drying the feet twice daily before applying the cream.

At the end of the study 28 out of the tolnaftate group, 11 out of the tea-tree group and seven from the placebo group had negative culture results (meaning there was no tinea pedis present).

This therefore shows that in this study tea-tree oil was more effective in reducing symptoms and tolnaftate was more effective in 'curing' the fungal infection. There were, however, some interesting points made in the 'Discussion' section of this paper. First, that a higher concentration of tea-tree oil might have resulted in an even more effective treatment for tinea pedis. Secondly that although credited with a higher cure rate (85%), there was evidence that tolnaftate had a minor skin irritant side effect on some of the patients.

Gout
A disease in which excess uric acid accumulates in the bloodstream and the joints. It often affects the big toe, which becomes red, hot, swollen and very painful. Besides dietary restrictions (especially on beer, organ meats and sugars) aromatherapy can help.
Aroma aid: Add juniper (4 drops), lemon and pine (2 each) to a bath. And increase the essential oil drops by 1 and mix in 20ml (⅔ fl oz) of base oil. Gently massage the aromatherapy blend *near* the gout-affected joint or area. Avoid the affected area, otherwise you may emit a loud scream!

Heartburn
See Chapter 5

High blood pressure
An increase in arterial blood pressure above the normal range (120/80). Cardiovascular problems, diet and stress are among the causes of high blood pressure. Always seek professional advice with this condition.
Aroma aid: I usually recommend the following blend to be used in conjunction with the allopathic medication that most hypertensive patients are taking. I have found that it is possible to effectively reduce blood pressure to an acceptable level using regular aromatherapy treatments. The effect can be instantaneous in some cases or the blood pressure may be slowly reduced over some months. In any case, the surprised doctor usually reduces the dosage of allopathic medication.

To a 50ml (1⅔ fl oz) base of almond oil add 12 drops of lavender, 7 of marjoram and 6 of ylang-ylang. Apply in a body massage weekly and 5ml in a bath. Stress can increase blood pressure and the 'anti-stress' action of these essential oils, along with their hypotensive properties, reduces the overall level of the blood pressure.

Heart Surgery Patients and Neroli

A randomised controlled trial involving 100 cardiac surgery patients was performed at the intensive care unit of Middlesex Hospital in the United Kingdom. The trial took five days and studied the effectiveness of neroli via a foot massage after cardiac surgery.

Method

The patients were divided into four groups:
- Nothing group: a control group with no communication for the 20-minute period after surgery.
- Chat group: a control group receiving only a casual 20-minute talk after surgery.
- Plain group: a group receiving a 20-minute foot massage with a plain vegetable oil (apricot kernel oil) after surgery.
- Aromatherapy group: a group receiving a 20-minute standardised foot massage using the neroli essential oil after surgery.

An independent recorder examined each group physiologically (measured heart rate, blood pressure and respiratory rate) and psychologically through a questionnaire (determining pain, anxiety, tension, calm, rest and relaxation).

Results

In this short study, no physiological benefits were found. However, the two groups receiving the foot massages experienced an improvement in their psychological well-being compared with the control groups. And the aromatherapy group experienced the most benefits from a reduction in anxiety mainly because of the oil's 'calming, relaxing and restful effects.'

High libido
When partners have differing sex drives, difficulties can arise in the relationship. Aromatherapy can be used to balance the sexual drives of both people in a relationship. If your sex drive is too high, try the anaphrodisiac mentioned below. (If it's too low, see the aphrodisiac blend under 'Impotence'.)
Aroma aid: Place 2 drops of marjoram on a tissue and inhale regularly. A massage with 5 drops of marjoram in 10ml of base oil twice weekly is also recommended.

Impotence
This condition may be more common than you think. Whenever I'm in a cab and I disclose my line of work, the driver always seems to ask about the remedy for impotence! Excessive alcohol, certain drugs, guilt or fear of failure, and certain illnesses may make it difficult to sustain an erection.
Aroma aid: Ylang-ylang, rose, patchouli, sandalwood and neroli are the essential oils indicated here. A once-weekly general body massage using 2 drops of any three of the above oils (make ylang-ylang one of them) in 10ml of base oil has proved beneficial in the treatment of impotence. The oriental herb ginseng can also assist this condition.

Male menopause
One explanation for male menopause (because it is not hormonal as with females) is that energy is more rapidly expended from the muscles with age — leading to tiredness. It is also suggested that fears of becoming old are involved.
Aroma aid: Lemongrass (1 drop), cedarwood (3 drops) and rosemary (4 drops), used in an aromatherapy burner or bath, can help in the treatment of the male menopause.

Migraine
See 'Headache', Chapter 5

Prostate disorders

Bacteria journeying from the bladder to the prostate can cause an infection in this gland. The inflammation can result in the prostate enlarging to a size greater than an orange. Symptoms include discomfort in the lower abdomen, frequent passing of urine with less volume and, in some cases, pain and discharge.

Aroma aid: Juniper, tea-tree and sandalwood essential oils have been found to be beneficial in the treatment of prostatitis. Using 4 drops of juniper, 3 of tea-tree and 2 of sandalwood, place a warm-to-hot compress over the lower abdomen. The oils can be added to a bath or used in a massage blend.

EASY 4-STEP BACK MASSAGE

Partners, family or friends will enjoy this easy 20-minute back rub. Always ensure your nails are short and clean when massaging. Tie your hair away from your face (if applicable).

Make or choose an aromatherapy massage blend and place 10ml in a small glass dish (for easy access). Ask the person receiving the massage to straddle a chair facing the back of it. You may need to place a pillow between the person's chest and chair. Alternatively, ask the person to lay on a bed or on cushions on the floor, if you don't have a massage table.

Roll a handtowel up (widthways) forming a horseshoe shape, and place it under the person's face (if they are lying down) to give the head support and to provide breathing room. As it is a back massage, the person may find it comfortable to rest their head to one side. Always ensure the room is warm and that the person is comfortable.

Tuck a bath towel into the top of the person's underwear, and if they are lying down, place a cotton blanket over their legs.

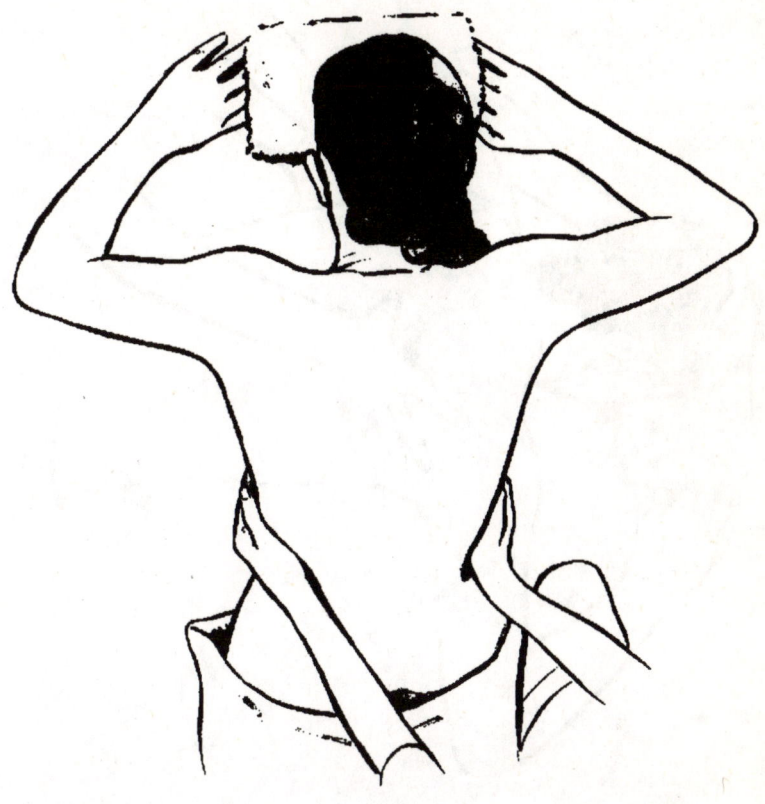

Step 1. With warm hands (rub them together before you apply the oil) apply sufficient oil to cover the back. Use firm, sweeping movements from the base of the spine to the shoulders and base of the neck and then move back down to the base of the spine.
If you are massaging a large or hairy male, you will need to apply more oil to allow a smooth massage.

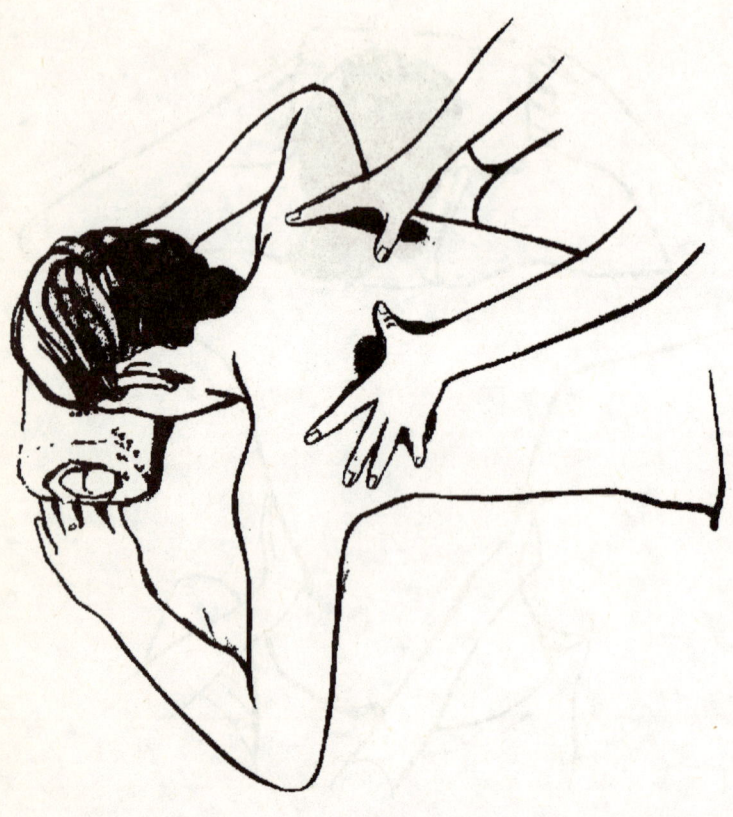

Step 2. Using small circular movements with the thumbs and starting at the base of the spine, travel up either side of the spine slowly and firmly. Ask the person if the pressure is right for them, and adjust it accordingly. Once at the base of the neck, with flat hands on the back, sweep across the shoulders and down to the base of the spine. Repeat this twice more.

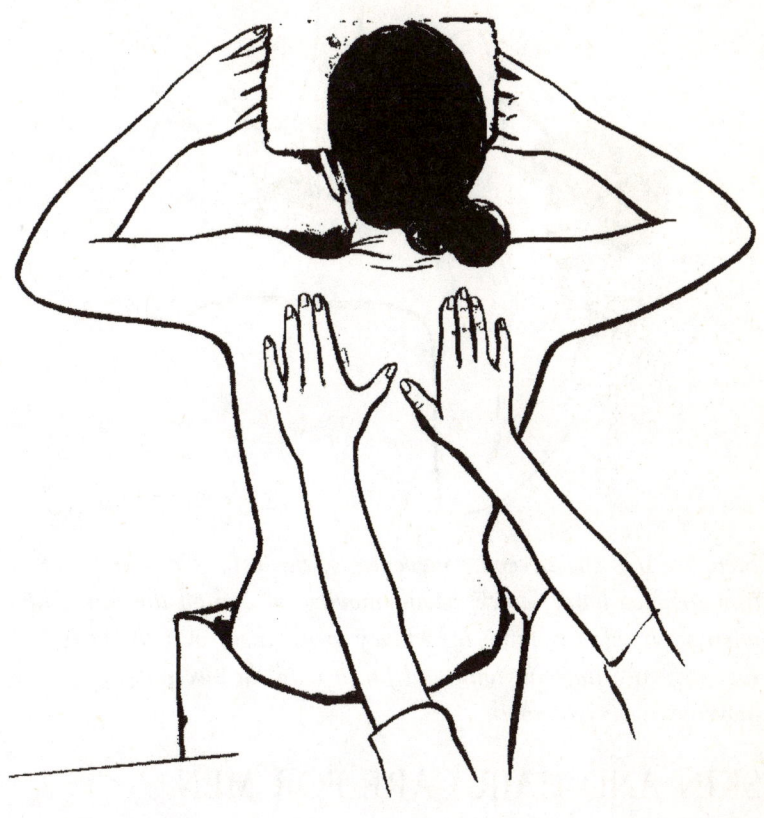

Step 3. Using a kneading action on the skin, slowly travel over the top of the buttock area, over the hips and all the way up to the shoulders. Repeat this twice more. Firm, sweeping movements up and down either side of the spine can follow each of the main movements.

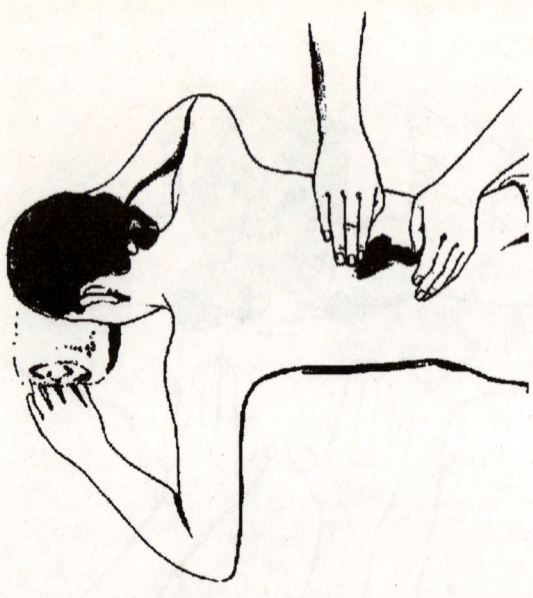

Step 4. After the sweeping movements, cup both hands and with a firm (not too hard), quick action, moving on and off the skin with alternate hands (avoiding the kidney area), move over the body. Do this three times in total and finish with the sweeping movements over the back.

SKIN AND HAIR CARE FOR MEN

Gone are the days when men were only supposed to use 'woody' aromas. Floral and fruity blends can also be very appealing and sexy for men.

An essential oil-enhanced soap or shower gel will not only clean but cater to your skin type. Use tea-tree oil for acned skin, sandalwood for dry skin, lemongrass for oily skin and lavender for normal skin.

AFTER SHOWER

There is now an abundance of aromatherapy-based deodorants on the market. Most contain the antibacterial tea-tree oil to combat body odour. Alternatively, try this do-it-yourself deodorant blend: mix 10 drops of lavender, 5 of sage, 5 of thyme and 10 of tea-tree oil with 2 tablespoons of vodka (and one nip for you!), then add half a cup of water. Place in a pump spray bottle and shake before use. The essential oils can be stirred into half a cup of cornflour for a powder deodorant. It's easy and effective.

If you have a favourite essential oil blend, place a small amount on a male's powerful pulse point — the spot just below the Adam's apple.

Now for the bane of most men's life — the morning shave. Aromatherapy can be of great use here:

- ➤ Soften the skin by applying a squeezed washer that has been soaked in a basin of warm-to-hot water and 7 drops of lavender oil. Leave the cloth on for at least 10 seconds, then repeat 2 or 3 times.
- ➤ Form a good lather with an aromatherapy-based foaming shave gel or soap. Using essential oils in your shaving routine can help to soothe the skin and prevent shaving rash.
- ➤ A non-alcohol based aftershave will avoid drying of the skin. Here is a simple aromatherapy blend that will tone, but won't sting your face. Mix 2 drops each of lavender, neroli and tea-tree into a third of a cup of purified or distilled water. Then get ready to splash it on.
- ➤ For men who suffer from shaving rash or chaffed skin, a replenishing moisturiser is essential. In addition, this blend will heal those sometimes unavoidable razor nicks — ouch.
To a base oil containing 5ml of wheatgerm oil, 10ml of avocado oil (both of these oils contain the skin-repairing vitamin E) and 25ml (about 1 fl oz) of sweet almond oil, add 8 drops of lavender, 7 of bergamot and 5 of sandalwood. Shake the blend and apply with the fingertips or cottonwool. The healing powers of chamomile would be of great use here, although it is quite expensive.

HAIR CARE

One of the most common male conditions, and one I am frequently asked advice about in the clinic, is balding. Unfortunately, Mr Hereditary has taken away any hope of a magic potion. But fortunately, aromatherapy has proven to be of assistance in reducing hair loss and improving the health of the scalp.

Lavender and rosemary are the key essential oils for hair loss. Mix 6 drops of lavender and 4 of rosemary into 20ml (⅔ fl oz) of jojoba or sweet almond oil. (Sage can be used to darken greying hair.)

AROMATHERAPY SCALP MASSAGE

This great massage will revive tired hair follicles and relax a tense scalp, stimulating hair growth and conditioning the scalp. Massaging the scalp will also bring fresh nutrients to the ailing hair follicles.

1. After shampooing the hair with a natural shampoo that is suited to your hair type, towel dry. Pour some oil onto the crown of the head, massaging it in with the thumbs on the temple and the fingers moving in a circular motion at the centre of the head.
2. Stroke the oil over the scalp from front to back, gently tugging or lifting the hair at the crown.
3. Apply more oil and, with kneading movements, slowly massage the entire head area.
4. Finish with stroking movements through the hair. Leave the oil in for 20 minutes and shampoo, or leave in overnight.

This massage can be repeated up to 4 times a week. For good results, continue for 6-8 weeks.

Chapter 7
AROMATHERAPY AND SPORT

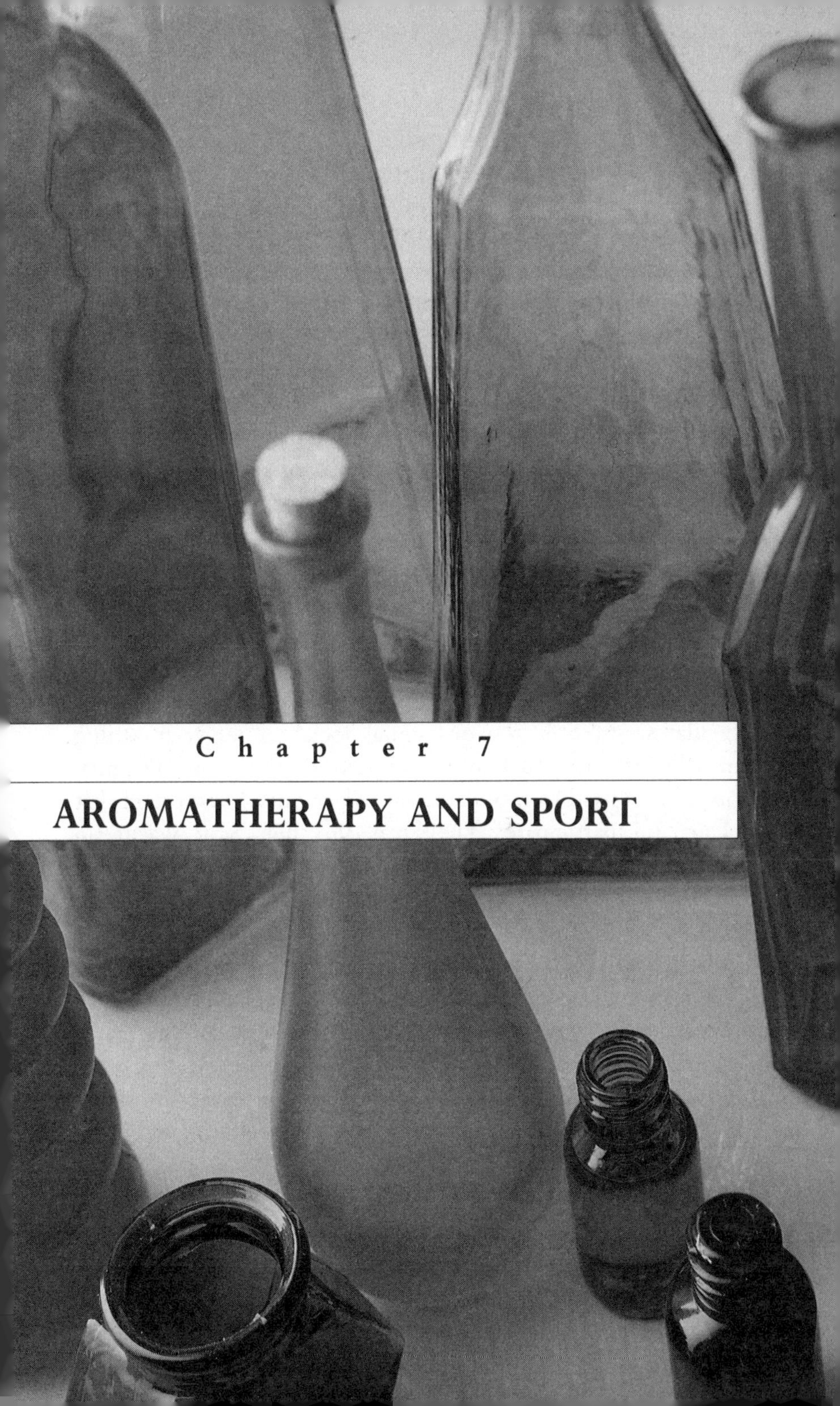

Is it stamina you need for that big race or game, concentration for good eye-to-ball co-ordination, a positive 'winning' attitude for competition, nerve calmers for risky adventure sport or practical sports medicine ideas? Aromatherapy can be a healthy partner in whichever sport you are involved with.

It's recommended that you do 20 minutes of exercise 3 times per week to maintain health. More exercise than this will certainly improve your fitness levels. People participate in sport for different reasons: some for fun, some for fitness and others for the adrenalin rush and sense of achievement. Let's look at the different types of sports — pleasure and fitness, adventure and competitive — to see how aromatherapy can help.

Pleasure and fitness sport: Walking, jogging, swimming, volleyball, squash, aerobics and golf are just some the sports people participate in for social reasons and to maintain their fitness levels. Some of these sports could also fit into the 'competition' group. If you're a person who doesn't participate in regular sport, only the occasional social game, your aching muscles will let you know at the end of the game. Essential oils can be used to motivate you to get out of bed or off that chair and participate. They can also help you warm up muscles and relieve aching ones.

Adventure sport: Skydiving, parachuting, bungie-jumping, rock-climbing and abseiling are all adventure sports. They give you that rush of excitement and boost your confidence — you did it, you climbed, jumped or glided where most mortals do not dare. Most adventurers will disclose not only determination but also a little anxiety or nervousness at times. Losing your nerve or concentration while participating in adventure sports is obviously not a good idea. The centring, calming and 'clear thinking' essential oils can help here.

Competitive sport: Basketball, tennis, football, netball, cricket, golf are competitive sports. Whether you're playing a one-off game or a series of matches, all you want to do is win and hopefully enjoy the game. Along with the team or player psychologist to psyche you up, think of another member of the team — aromatherapy. Essential oils can help you to develop a 'winning' frame of mind, giving you confidence and motivation. Plus they can increase your strength and stamina or, if a ball is involved in the sport, your co-ordination.

Whatever your sporting interest, there is an aromatherapy blend for your physical or mental/emotional support.

AROMATHERAPY PHYSICAL SUPPORT

ACHES AND PAINS

For general aches and pains after sport, a bath using pine, juniper and rosemary is recommended. Place 4 drops of juniper and 2 each of pine and rosemary into a running bath. You'll feel the relieving effect very soon.

BRUISING

Gently apply neat lavender to the bruise, then apply the homoeopathic remedy arnica 30x to assist healing. This may need to be repeated 3 times daily, depending on the size of the bruise.

COOL-DOWN SPRAY

To help you to cool down and fight fatigue, or sometimes exhaustion, make up a spray of peppermint.

In a stainless-steel or glass spray bottle, add 10 drops of peppermint to half a litre of filtered water. Shake and apply the spray to the face and body, holding the bottle 20–30cm away.

Cramping

Besides sucking on a 'neuromuscular' magnesium phosphate tablet straight away to ease the cramp, rub the area with a blend of lavender, cypress and rosemary. It's usually the calf muscles that spasm.

Add 5 drops of lavender, 3 drops of cypress and 2 drops of rosemary to 20ml (⅔ fl oz) of sweet almond oil. Work the blend into the affected muscle with warm hands, working up the muscle. This will provide quick relief.

Influenza

Athletes can be more prone to a cold or flu than a person of lesser fitness. I have heard of top athletes 'disappearing' from sight when someone sneezes near them. They will go to great lengths to avoid a performance-inhibiting infection.

If you feel a cold coming on, besides taking vitamin C or garlic and echinacea supplements, try an aromatherapy 'anti-flu' steam inhalation. Place 2 drops of eucalyptus, tea-tree and lemon into a medium-sized bowl of hot water. Place a towel over your head and inhale for a minute or so. You may need to repeat this in a few hours.

Muscle Tone

You don't have to be a 'Mr or Ms Universe' to participate in sport. However, good muscle tone is important. A diet high in protein and low in fat, along with regular exercise, will assist in building muscle tone. Essential oils can be regularly massaged into the muscles to improve their tone.

Add juniper (6 drops) and rosemary (4 drops) to 20ml (⅔ fl oz) of sweet almond oil. Massage the blend into the specific area twice weekly.

Perspiration and Odour

Sweating is a healthy excretion of the fluids and toxins that are within the body. It is increased during sporting activities and can produce an unpleasant odour. Natural deodorants aim to reduce the bacteria that surround the sweat glands and produce the odour. A spray made from filtered water and the essential oils of tea-tree, lemongrass and cypress can help to decrease odour and perspiration.

Place 5 drops of cypress and 3 each of tea-tree and 2 of lemongrass into a stainless-steel or glass spray bottle containing half a litre of water. Shake before use and apply under the arms.

Sprains and Strains

Land the wrong way and a sprain or strain may be inevitable. Besides the usual first aid of ice, compression and elevation, an aromatherapy compress can alleviate pain, swelling and discomfort.

A cold compress of lavender (4 drops) plus marjoram and pine (2 drops each) applied regularly is indicated here.

Stamina

Lemongrass is one of the most energising essential oils. Place a few drops on a tissue and inhale. A peppermint and water spray can also fight fatigue. The herb ginseng is used as a supplement by some athletes to improve their stamina.

Warm-up Muscle Rub

To warm the muscles and improve circulation, try the following blend. To 50ml (1⅔ fl oz) of a sweet almond base oil add 12 drops of lavender, 8 drops of rosemary and 5 drops of eucalyptus. This blend is best applied to the legs in an upward sweeping motion.

Sports Leg Massage

During sport and training our legs do a lot of work. The muscles can become tight and store acid wastes (that are a by-product of muscular activity), making them ache. Next, I'll explain how to massage the legs and feet with a detoxifying, anti-ache aromatherapy blend.

Step 1. Ask the sports player to leave their shirt and underpants on and lie on a towel-covered massage table. Ensure the room is warm and cover their back and buttocks area with a towel or cotton blanket. Make the person comfortable.
Step 2. Add the essential oils of lavender (5 drops), juniper (3 drops) and rosemary (2 drops) to 20ml of sweet almond oil. Blend well and place 5–10ml in a small glass dish.
Step 3. With firm, sweeping movements with the flat of your hand, apply the oil up the body from the feet to the sides and tops of the legs. Repeat all movements 3 times.

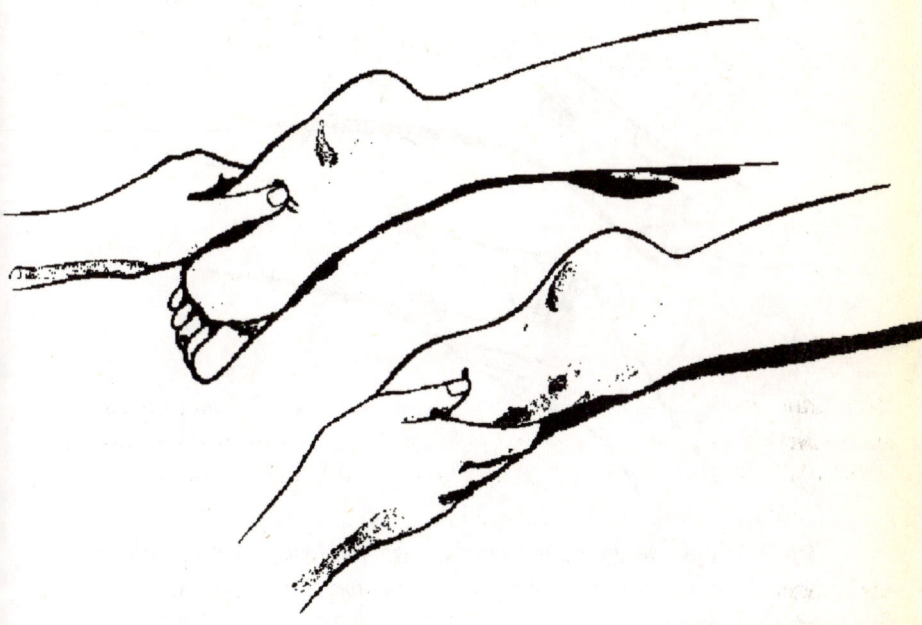

Step 4. Using both hands, work on both feet and legs simultaneously. Start at the ball of each foot with small circular thumb movements and move slowly up the foot to the heel. If you feel any 'crystal-like' substance below the skin, spend a little extra time to gently dissolve them.

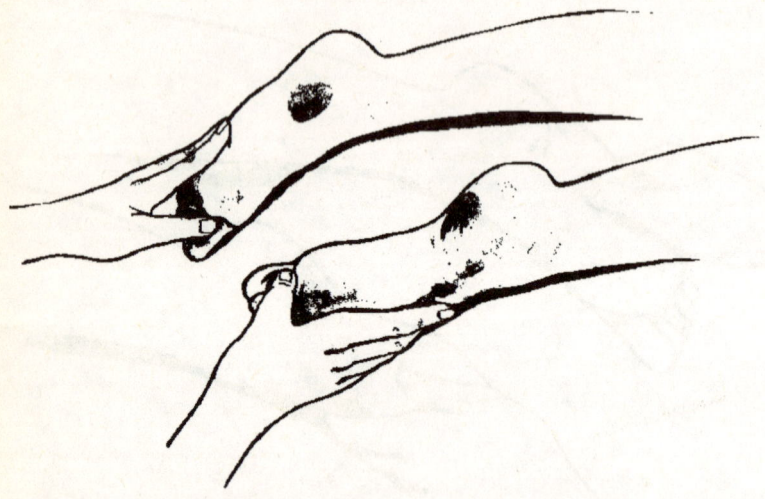

Step 5. Apply sweeping movements over the foot and end with gentle thumb pressures to the pad of each toe (using the pad of your thumb).
Step 6. Slowly slide your thumb in short, firm, side-ways movements over the foot from the ball to the heel. Ensure that you cover the whole foot.

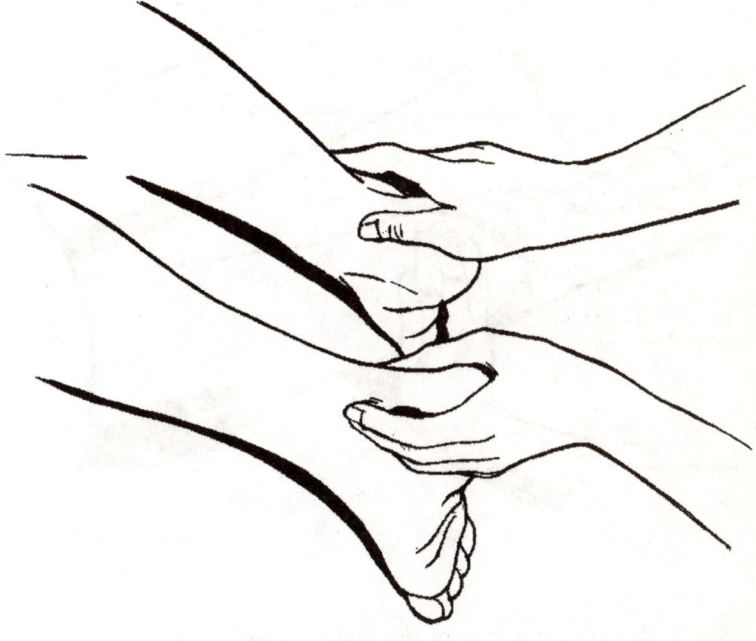

Step 7. With the thumb to one side of the ankle and the fingers to the other, gently rub (moving slowly back and forth). Do five of these movements.

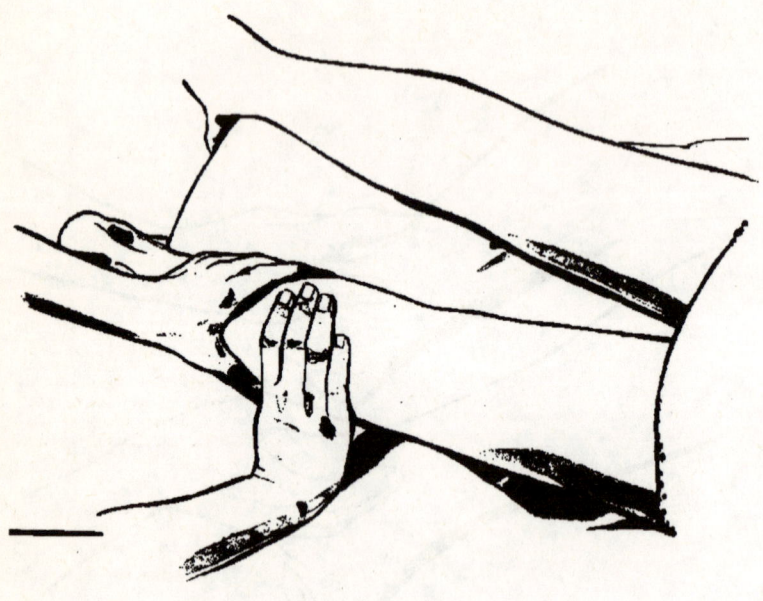

Step 8. Move to one side of the table. Travel up the legs, kneading the calf muscles and the tops of the legs. This movement can be alternated with firm, large semi-circular-shaped movements up the legs.
Step 9. Apply slow, firm sweeping movements up the feet and legs. (optional)

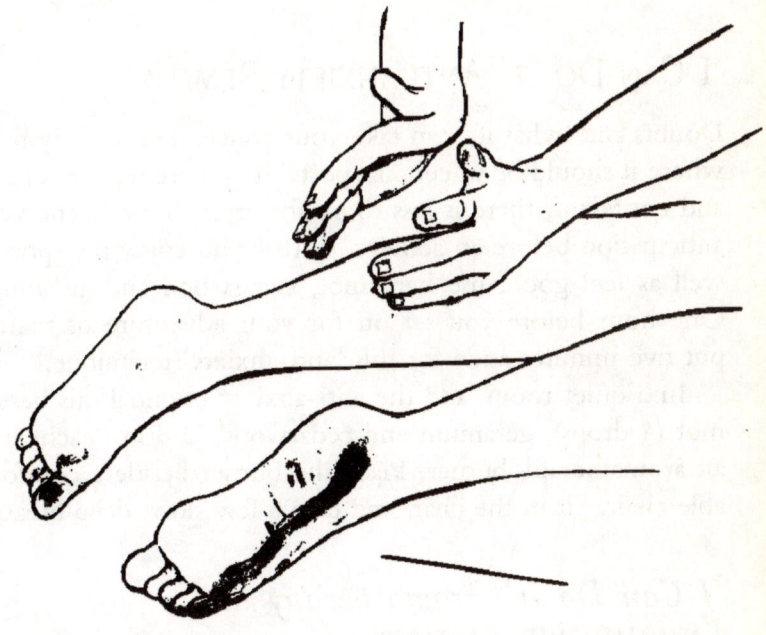

Step 10. Using both hands and a gentle but firm chopping action, travel from the calf muscle (missing the knees) and onto the top of the leg. Repeat the action on the other leg. Standing at the feet, finish the leg and foot massage with three sweeping movements up the feet and legs (allow the pressure to ease after each movement).

AROMATHERAPY MENTAL AND EMOTIONAL SUPPORT

'I Can Do It' Anti-anxiety Remedy

Doubts and 'what ifs' can take your concentration away from where it should be in certain sports. If you are feeling relaxed and confident, there is less room for error. To calm nervous anticipation before an activity, so that you enjoy the sport as well as feel good, use bergamot, cedarwood and geranium. One hour before you set off for your adventure or match, put five minutes aside for this 'anti-anxiety' technique.

In a quiet room, add the anti-anxiety essential oils bergamot (4 drops), geranium and cedarwood (2 drops each) into an aromatherapy burner. Place the burner beside a comfortable chair. Sit in the chair and take a few slow, deep breaths.

'I Can Do It' Aromatherapy and Visualisation Exercise

With every breath of the aromatherapy blend you take you can feel the tension in your muscles unwinding and letting go. Count backwards from 5 to 1.
5 ... you can feel any tension in your head, neck and shoulder muscles draining out and drifting away from your body.
4 ... any tension in your shoulders, arms and hands is draining out through your fingers.
3 ... you can feel your chest, abdomen and back relaxing more and more with every breath you take.
2 ... any tension in your buttocks, hip and thigh muscles is draining away from your body.
1 ... your body is feeling very, very calm and very relaxed. Any tension is draining out of your legs and feet. You are completely relaxed.

Visualise or think of your sport today. See yourself confidently and successfully achieving your goal. You know you can achieve it. It's yours. You've done it. See other people congratulating you. You can even hear other people talking among themselves, discussing your achievement.

Gradually and slowly, become aware of your circulation, start to move your hands and toes. Begin to stretch and feel the flow of energy and vitality running through your body. You are relaxed, calm and confident of success. When you're ready, open your eyes.

Concentration

Many sports require total concentration, especially in the competitive and adventure arenas. Mental fatigue may creep into your game, if you are not prepared. Basil and rosemary are the prime essential oils that are indicated here. Place 2 drops of each onto a cottonwool ball or tissue and inhale regularly before the activity.

Negative Attitude

One negative player in a team can have a domino effect on the other players. In a one-person activity, it can be just as damaging.

Inhaling a few drops of clary sage or chamomile from a tissue or cottonwool ball will help to keep you positive.

Sore Losers

Sore losers can often dump their frustrations onto the people who are close to them or onto their opponents. If they are not prepared to do something about it, subtly place 2 drops of rose, ylang-ylang and chamomile in an aromatherapy burner nearby. Sit back and watch the change!

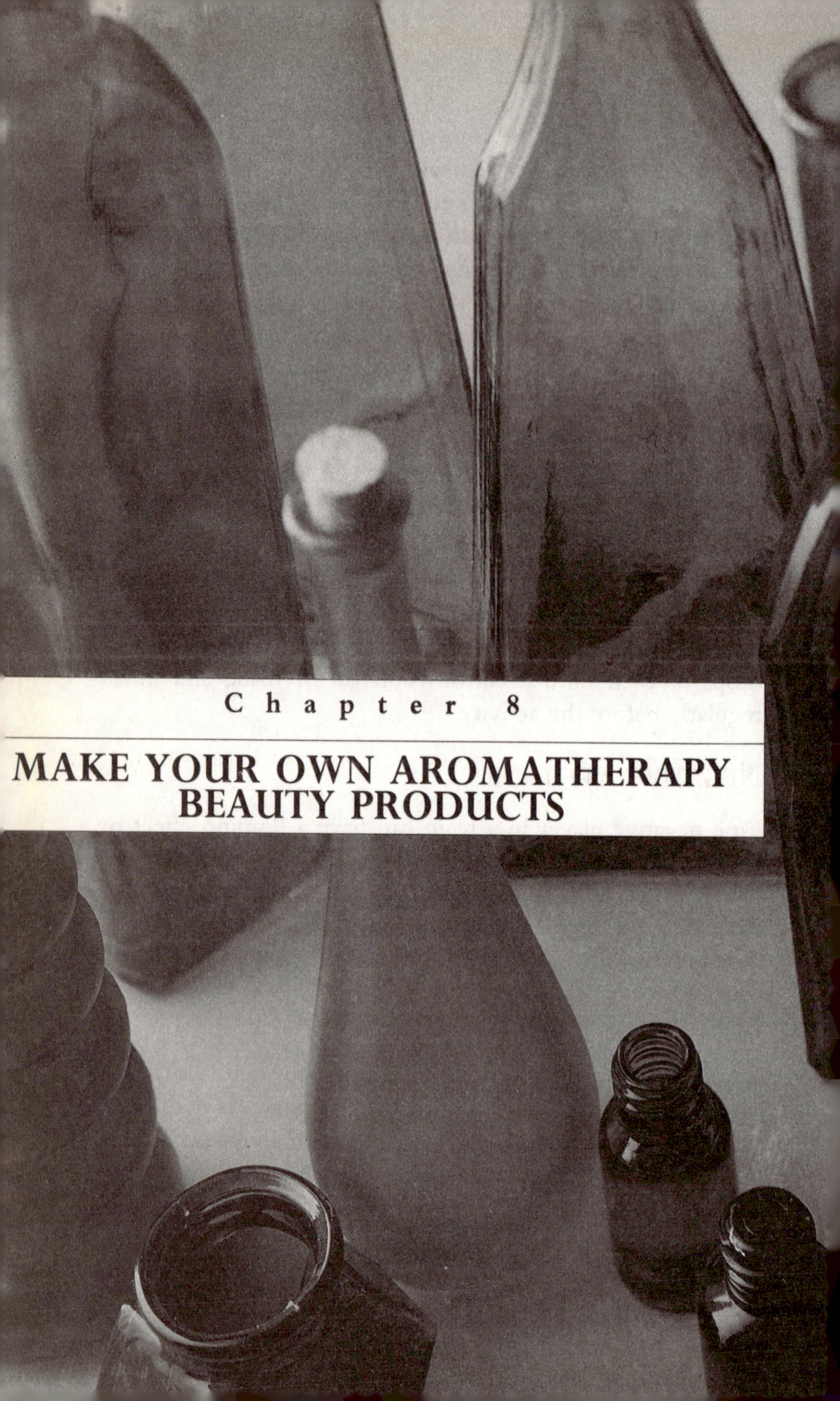

Chapter 8
MAKE YOUR OWN AROMATHERAPY BEAUTY PRODUCTS

Thank goodness we don't live in Elizabethan times. Some of their beauty products had unfortunate side-effects, such as discoloured and scaly skin, decayed and blackened teeth! Unlike the Egyptians, who used essential oils to stay young and red ochre for a pink colouring, Englishwomen used red crystalline mercuric sulphide. And the popular whitened-skin look was achieved by mixing white lead with vinegar!

In modern times there is a demand for safe, affordable, natural beauty products. The aim of natural beauty products is not to create a multicoloured facade to inspire awe in others, it is about enhancing the quality and vitality of an individual's skin, hair and nails. Feeling good about ourselves on the inside also shines through to the outside.

Essential oils are exceptional beauty aids. They provide rejuvenating and therapeutic properties for radiant skin but also have a positive influence on how we feel. Frowning is a good example of how our emotions can affect our appearance. Worry lines do not take long to take hold. Essential oils can uplift, calm, balance and energise the mind and emotions. Imagine a beauty cream or lotion that gets rid of your pimples or dry skin and helps you to feel good too! I know, 'Where do I get them?', you're saying.

Effective, good-quality beauty products can be made at home. In a few simple steps you can make aromatherapy cleansers, toners, moisturisers and masques to suit your skin type. Make a batch and try it; you'll be surprised at the difference in your complexion.

First of all, why natural?

WHY NATURAL?

The alternatives to natural essential oils are synthetic 'nature identicals'. These are used extensively throughout the perfume and flavouring industries. Nature identicals are much cheaper than natural oils but they can have undesirable side-effects if used therapeutically.

There are hundreds of constituents in an essential oil, and nature identicals can not exactly copy them. They are said to be 96 per cent accurate. Vital energy and natural constituents contained within rose petals, lavender heads or the wood of sandalwood, for instance, will not be found in these synthetic substitutes. If you're serious about aromatherapy and want the best for your beauty routine, choose 100 per cent pure essential oils.

Now let's find out more about how essential oils benefit the skin and how easy it is to diagnose your skin type.

AROMATHERAPY SKIN CARE

Essential oils have many characteristics that are ideal for maintenance, repair and replenishment of the skin.

How Essential Oils Benefit the Skin

Action	Benefit to Skin Type	Essential Oil
Anti-allergic	Reduces hypersensitivity reactions common to dry skin	Chamomile, rose
Anti-inflammatory	Reduces inflammation of dry or oily, acned skin	Clary sage, frankincense, geranium, orange, sandalwood, tea-tree
Antibacterial	Destroys bacteria common to oily skin	Most oils, in particular lemongrass, tea-tree, thyme

Anti-oxidant	Prevents deterioration or ageing of skin	Lemongrass, rosemary, thyme
Antisebaceous	Reduces the production of sebum (oil) from sweat glands common to oily skin	Clary sage, rosemary
Antiseptic	Destroys microbes common to oily skin	Most oils
Astringent	Tightens the skin, assisting oily skin particularly	Clary sage, cypress, frankincense, geranium, lemon, lemongrass, patchouli, rosemary, thyme
Cell regeneration	Stimulates new cell growth important for mature skin	Lavender, neroli
Circulation stimulant	Brings nutrients to the tissues, improving tone and health for all skin types	Cypress, geranium, lemon, lemongrass, neroli, rose, rosemary, thyme
Detoxifier	Increases elimination of potentially harmful substances from the body, assists congested skin	Juniper, lemon, lavender, patchouli, thyme
Scar healing	Heals scar tissue	Lavender primarily

Which Skin Type Are You?

The first step in helping your skin with aromatherapy is to identify your skin type. Is it oily, combination, normal or dry? Once this has been diagnosed the essential oils that suit your particular skin type can be chosen.

Skin types and your face

Skin type	Characteristics	Essential oils
Oily	Large, open pores Shiny surface Pimples with black or white heads present Acne may be present	Clary Sage, juniper, lemon, lemongrass, rosemary, tea-tree, thyme
Combination	Oily forehead, nose and chin (T-zone) Cheeks may be normal to dry	Choose oils from the list above and below
Normal	Fine texture No open pores or dry patches Pimples rarely present	Chamomile, geranium, lavender, patchouli, rose, sandalwood
Dry-Mature	Can appear tight May have dry, flaky patches Broken capillaries may be present Lined and wrinkled Can be highly sensitive and allergic	Chamomile, frankincense, geranium, lavender, neroli, patchouli, rose, sandalwood, ylang-ylang

Back to Basics

Come on, hands up those who sometimes skip the twice-daily beauty basics of cleansing, toning and moisturising? Or what about those on the run who skip the toner or dash for the splash of soap and water (my hand's up)? Sticking to a proper beauty routine takes a conscious effort. But, just as paying attention to a balanced diet, exercise, rest and attitude is important for health and vitality, so is our attention to hygiene and skin care. Understanding the rationale behind the need for each step of our regular beauty work outs may give it more meaning and motivation for you.

Step 1: Cleanse

The skin is the largest eliminative organ in the body. Waste products can therefore be transported and dumped onto the skin's surface. Add to this the external bombardment of the skin by petrol fumes, pollution or grit, and you can see why clean, clear pores are necessary to prevent the build-up of toxins on or in the skin. Lacklustre skin, pimples and blackheads can be the result. We clean our teeth daily to prevent plaque build-up, so why not our face?

- Add no more than 6 drops (in total) of essential oils, selecting from your skin type list, to a warm basin of water. Soak a washer in your aromatherapy blend, squeeze it and wipe over the face. This removes surface grit and dead skin cells.
- Another option is to place a few drops of the essential oil into your favourite natural cleanser or use a gentle soap that contains essential oils for your skin type.

Step 2: Tone

Toning removes excess cleanser, closes the pores and improves circulation to the skin. It is a vital middle step in a good beauty program. Aromatherapy is well suited to filling this role.

Dry skin toner: Rose water or neroli water
Sensitive skin toner: Chamomile water

Normal/Combination skin toner: Lavender water or any of the above
Oily skin toner: Lemongrass water

Make your own aromatherapy toner

The toners need to be stored in a dark glass bottle in a cool place. They will last around 4–6 weeks. As an optional extra you can place 2 drops of the relevant essential oils into the toner.

Rose toner

Place 2 cups of rose petals into a medium-sized bowl and cover with boiling water. Place a lid on the bowl, allow the water to cool, then strain. Repeat this procedure using the boiled rose water.

Chamomile toner

Place 2 chamomile teabags into 2 cups (500ml/16 fl oz) of boiled water, then cover until cool.

Lavender water

Put 20 fresh lavender flower heads in a bowl and cover with boiling water. Place the lid on the bowl, allow the water to cool, then strain. Repeat using the boiled lavender water.

Lemongrass water

Place 2 lemongrass teabags into 2 cups (500ml/16 fl oz) of boiled water, then cover until cool.

Moisten a cottonwool pad with the aromatherapy toner and wipe over the face, taking care to avoid the eye area.

Step 3: Moisturise

As a baby our skin contains nearly 90 per cent moisture, but as we grow older, alas, we lose much of this. Our moisture content can be down as low as 10 per cent by the time we reach 40 or 50! Wind, air-conditioning, dry climates or overheated rooms can rob our skin of moisture. A moisturiser is necessary to plump the skin and to prevent you from looking like a prune.

Pick two essential oils from your skin type list and place 3 drops in total into 5g or 5ml of either of the bases below. Although we're dealing with small amounts here, use the blending factors and notes as a guide (see Chapter 9). It's obvious that if blending for oily skin, 1 drop of lemongrass would be used to perhaps 2 of tea-tree oil. For normal skin, use 1 drop of patchouli to 2 drops of lavender, and for dry, perhaps use 1 drop of rose to 2 of sandalwood.

Skin type	Base Blend
Dry-sensitive	15ml (½ fl oz) apricot kernel oil + 5ml avocado oil + 2ml evening primrose oil
Normal-oily	15ml (½ fl oz) apricot or peach kernel oil + 5ml wheatgerm oil

Fragrant facial cream

Aromatherapy companies now manufacture an odourless base cream, a natural alternative to Sorbolene cream and other mineral oil-based products. I use this cream extensively for facials and therapeutic applications in the clinic. Buy some from your aromatherapy stockist and add the essential oils for your skin type. Or make your own facial cream — it's easy!

Slowly add 20ml (⅔ fl oz) of sweet almond oil and 10g of beeswax to a double saucepan (with water in the bottom pan) that is placed on low heat. A heat-resistant bowl in a pot of water will also do. Stir continuously until well blended.

Remove the saucepan from the heat and gradually add up to 20ml

(⅔ fl oz) of purified water, blending well until the mixture is creamy. Allow to cool slightly and add 15 drops of your skin type's essential oils (in total).

Place the mixture in a container and store in the refrigerator or in a cool place.

Use the same recipe for a body lotion, only add more purified water until the consistency you desire has been reached.

Blend and place in a dark bottle in a cool place. Shake well before use.

OTHER SKIN TREATMENTS

Steam

An aromatherapy steam will send therapeutic vapours into your open pores. Look at the actions and benefits list of essential oils previously mentioned, and tailor a steam treatment to suit your skin's needs.

Blackheads: Do you have a few blackheads or does your skin feel oily and congested? Try juniper (3 drops) and thyme (2 drops) in a medium-sized bowl of hot water.

Blackheads form if fatty material, sebum and keratin, remain in the pore. The pore's surface becomes black when the keratin oxidises. Both oils will detoxify and thyme, being antibacterial, anti-oxidant and astringent, will kill the bacteria, prevent oxidation of keratin and shrink the blackhead to allow for easy removal.

To remove a blackhead, use a blackhead remover (that's a bit obvious), usually available from pharmacies. Alternatively, place a tissue around both index fingers and gently squeeze. Swab the cleansed pore with the thyme water mixture to close it.

Dry-mature skin: This type of skin tends to have more wrinkles. Imagine the benefits of using the 'anti-ageing' or rejuvenating essential oils of neroli (2 drops) and lavender (3 drops) in a steam.

Exfoliate

By exfoliating you are removing the build-up of dead cells from the skin's surface. If you don't remove them regularly (2 or 3 times weekly for oily skin and once weekly for dry-normal skin), the pores can choke on the refuse. It's a bit like remembering to take the garbage out on Sunday nights; if you forget, the rubbish will pile up.

There are some terrific natural exfoliants available that contain gentle agents such as oatmeal. Read the label to check that it is a natural product and add 2 drops of your skin type's essential oil to the exfoliant before using.

Aromatherapy masques

In my workshops part of the practical session involves making your own face masque to take home. It's great fun. It reminds me of making mud pies as a little girl, except the clay is going into a jar, not a pretend oven.

I recommend being adventurous when deciding on the ingredients for your face masque. Kaolin or 'Fullers Earth' is the standard clay used. Besides this, I have discovered some green, red, pink, yellow and white clays under the 'Argiletz' label that are perfect for masques. Generally, clay draws out impurities from the skin, giving a deep cleanse. In addition, each 'Argiletz' clay has its own benefits for the skin:

Green clay: For tissue repair. This is the most effective toxin-drawing clay. It is healing, antiseptic, cleansing and anti-inflammatory. Indicated for normal to oily skin.

Red clay: Is high in iron oxide and helpful for broken capillaries and bags under the eyes. It is good for muscle toning. Indicated for skin with broken capillaries.

Pink clay: Improves skin softness. It disinfects and heals because of the trace elements it contains (calcium, iron, magnesium, phosphorus, silicon and sodium). Fragile, dehydrated skin can benefit from the use of pink clay. It is also ideal for tissue firming, particularly for the bust, thighs and buttocks. Indicated for dry, mature or sensitive skin.

White clay: This may be used as a hair pack by mixing it with water prior to shampooing. It will alleviate dry scalp disorders as well as greasy hair problems. Also indicated for dry-sensitive skin.

Yellow clay: Particularly good for sun-damaged skin. It is rich in calcium, iron, magnesium, phosphorus, potassium and silicon.

Other natural beauty components of a masque could include:

Yoghurt: Is soothing and nutritive to the skin.

Honey: Is healing, soothing and a natural preservative.

Strawberries*: Whitens the skin to remove freckles, and is good for sensitive or sunburnt skin. The juice has antibacterial properties and can be helpful for pimply skin.

Stewed apple*: Traditionally used for skin inflammation. It is good for dry, allergic or pimply and acned skin.

*You can use fresh strawberries or stewed apple you make yourself (without the sugar). Another equally beneficial option is to buy sugar-free pureed strawberry and apple combinations from the supermarket.

Make your own masque

Using the previous information as a guide, formulate an aromatherapy beauty masque suitable to your skin type.

Fruit and flower masque

Add 1 crushed strawberry or 1 flat teaspoon of apple or fruit puree to 1 tablespoon of yoghurt*. Blend in well with a fork.

Add 1 teaspoon of clay and mix thoroughly.

Choose from two or three essential oils from your skin type list and add 5-8 drops in total. Mix well.

Place the masque in an airtight jar and refrigerate.

*A small quantity of a nourishing base oil such as evening primrose oil and/or avocado oil can replace the yoghurt.

This will last you for three masques, enough for one per week. Recycle the jar for your next masque treatment.

Water, clay and essential oil masque

Select the clay and essential oils for your skin type. Place 1 tablespoon of clay into a small mixing dish. Add enough filtered water to make a smooth paste.
Add the essential oils (5-8 drops) and stir into the clay paste.
Including a mashed strawberry and lemon oil (2 drops) with the 'skin' essential oil patchouli (3 drops) in a masque may help to fade pigmentations of the skin. A naturopath can also help with herbal remedies internally.

To use your masque:
1. Cleanse and tone your skin.
2. Brush on or smooth on your aromatherapy cleansing and healing masque. Soft, thick brushes are available from pharmacies, department stores or beauty suppliers. Leave the masque on for up to 20 minutes.
3. Remove with a warm, wet washer.
4. Moisturise your face with a suitable aromatherapy cream.

Aromatherapy Hair Care

You can tell a lot about a person's health by looking at their hair. Is it shiny and bouncy or limp and lustreless? Does it look like a white Christmas from the dandruff? Is the hair greying surprisingly quickly or falling out unexpectedly?

Although the hair itself is dead, nourishing and stimulating the scalp can improve the condition of new hair growth. A balanced wholefood diet, regular exercise and stress-management techniques are all crucial for maintaining healthy hair. The scalp needs to receive a good supply of blood so that the 'hair' nutrients — zinc, B complex vitamins and silica — reach the hair follicles.

HAIR AND SHOCK

You've probably heard tales of shock victims' hair turning grey or white. Imagine the benefits of inhaling the crisis or shock essential oil neroli, or taking the Bach Flower emergency blend called Rescue Remedy at this time. It may even prevent the dramatic colour change.

HAIR AND STRESS

When I first graduated from naturopathic college I worked part-time for a leading natural health and beauty company. I was employed to 'woman' the naturopathic 'hotline' and answer the public's, practitioners' and health food/pharmacy stores' queries about the products and general natural health. I kept a daily tally of the calls I received (around 80) and the subject of the enquires. The most common ailment I was asked advice about was alopecia, or hair loss, in women!

After obtaining basic details, it seemed the common link between all the calls was stress. Stress can deplete our body of B vitamins and zinc, healthy hair nutrients. The anti-stress essential oils of bergamot, lavender, orange and sandalwood, for instance, can also help to reduce hair loss by supporting the nervous system.

HAIR LOSS: JOAN'S STORY

I would like to tell you about this 'hair loss' case history because I truly found it fascinating.

When Joan first came to me she was suffering from alopecia. She was 37 and already had whitish-grey hair. Joan started to question her symptoms when her hair began to fall out in bundles (I mean *bundles*) when she combed or brushed it. I went through Joan's health and lifestyle history. There was a stressful situation at work with a co-worker, but nothing she couldn't handle. Her diet was full of wholefoods and she was drinking lots of water. She walked four times each week for 30 minutes at a time, and she appeared to have a calm and easygoing outlook on life.

Treatment

I prescribed a complex supplement that contained B vitamins, zinc and the hair mineral silica. I gave Joan a head and scalp massage using juniper, lavender and rosemary in a base of apricot kernel oil/jojoba oil. I then gave her a 50ml (1⅔ fl oz) blend and instructed her to massage it into her scalp 2 or 3 times per week initially, before she went to bed. To assist the oils to penetrate the scalp, she was to apply a warmed towel for 10 minutes. She was instructed to wash the blend out of her hair in the morning's shower or bath.

When Joan came to see me again after two weeks, her condition had only improved slightly. I was not happy with her progress and ordered a hair mineral analysis test for her hair. This is a simple test in which a few tufts of hair (from the back of the neck area) are assessed for their mineral composition. The amazing test results answered the 'why?' about the slow-healing hair loss problem.

Joan's copper levels were sky-high, and copper is a mineral that competes with zinc for absorption in the body. On further questioning Joan about her plumbing at home and work, I discovered that she had copper water pipes connected to her home and the hot-water urn at work contained copper. I strongly recommended that she purchase a good-quality water filter for home and a portable one for work, which she did. I massaged her again with the same blend and increased the amount of zinc she was taking for the short term.

Two weeks later the problem had cleared!

Different Hair Types

Matching hair types and essential oils

Hair type	Characteristics	Essential oils
Oily	Excessive oiliness May have dry ends May lack lustre	Bergamot, cypress, lavender, rosemary
Normal	Not dry or oily Shiny appearance	Geranium, lavender, sandalwood
Dry and damaged	Split ends Fly-away hairs Lacks lustre	Frankincense, geranium, lavender, patchouli

Shampoo: Add 2 drops of an essential oil for your hair type into a natural shampoo (1 wash quantity).

If dandruff is a problem, make a blend of lavender (5 drops), rosemary (3 drops) and cedarwood (2 drops) in 10ml each of jojoba and sweet almond oil. Apply to the scalp twice weekly.

Hair rinse: Rinses can add shine and a mild, almost seducing aroma to the hair. To make a rinse to use after a shampoo and condition, add 4–6 drops of essential oils to 0.5–1 litre (16–32 fl oz) of water. Wash through the hair and leave to dry naturally.

To lighten or darken hair and to add shine, see Chapter 4.

NAILS

Nails are an important way of measuring health. Do your nails have any of the following symptoms:
- numerous vertical lines?
- faint or heavy horizontal ridges?
- flaky skin around the edges?
- a blue/purple colour at their base?

Vertical lines

Can mean that you 'run off your nerves'. Most people have these lines, but if the lines are deeply ridged, you must take quick action to restore and strengthen your nervous system. The anti-stress essential oils, especially lavender and sandalwood regularly used in a massage blend, are indicated here.

Horizontal ridges

The nail takes six months to grow from the base of the nail to the top (excluding the white nail area at the top). If a deep horizontal ridge is present, it can indicate that your mental, physical or emotional state was deleteriously affected six months ago. If it is halfway between the base and the top of the nail, you will know that the illness occurred three months ago. Although this is past information, with a marked indication like this the systems of the body may still be suffering. Use the appropriate essential oils to aid the healing process.

Flaky skin around the nails

This common sign can indicate that you are lacking in B group vitamins (found in wholegrains, cereals and yeast). It usually means that either your diet is lacking in B vitamin-containing foods or you are under stress. Again, the anti-stress essential oils can heal. Another suggestion is to make a blend of apricot kernel oil (5ml) and wheatgerm (2ml) with 3 drops of lavender. Apply this to the cuticle and edges of the nail to heal and nourish.

Blue/purple colour at the base

A colouring of this type can indicate poor circulation. Regular exercise and a general massage using 3 drops of rosemary, 5 drops of geranium and 2 drops of eucalyptus in 20ml (⅔ fl oz) of a base oil will improve this condition.

To strengthen your nails, see Chapter 4.

Chapter 9
A–Z GUIDE TO ESSENTIAL OILS

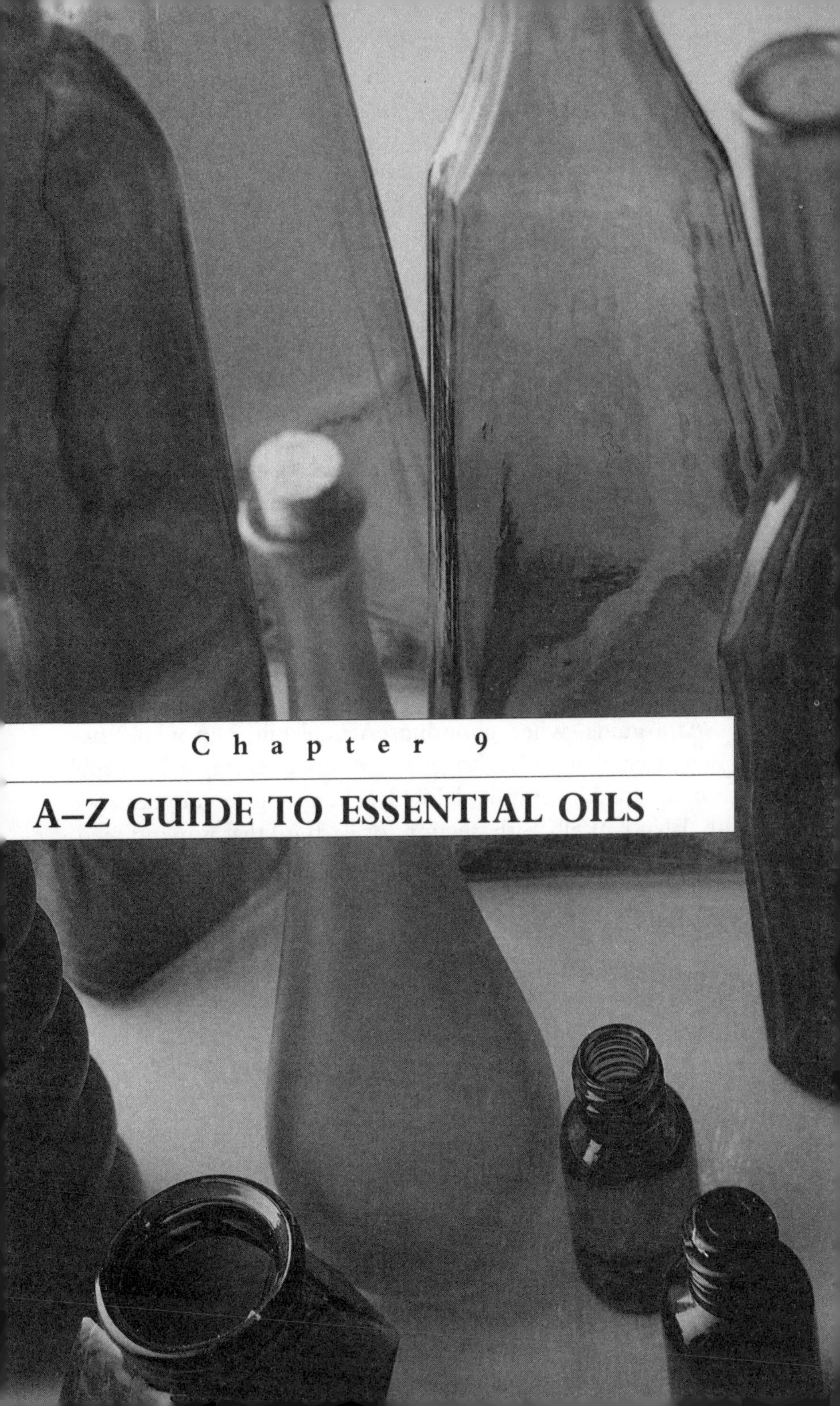

The common essential oils set out below can be found in most health food stores, pharmacies and gift stores. Before we discuss these oils individually, how to blend essential oils will be covered. It will give the individual oils more practical meaning.

BLENDING ESSENTIAL OILS

Odours are very personal. What one person loves, another may find intolerable. As a general rule, always follow your nose. Is the blend pleasant to you? Even when working towards a therapeutic outcome it's still important that the blend is not offensive to you or, more specifically, to the recipient of the blend. A good example of this is the 'tranquillity' essential oil vetiver. To me it smells like a swamp, but I could not leave it out of an insomnia formula. So I improve the blend's odour with lavender or geranium.

As a guide, when choosing essential oils, you would not put extreme opposites together. A good example is deeply relaxing frankincense and highly energising lemongrass. See the 'Blends Well With' section for each oil that is mentioned. You can blend essential oils outside of this list, but make sure they have a good synergy. To test this, place a drop of each oil onto paper strips and wave them under your nose. Are they pleasant or do they fight each other?

Next choose your base oil. The 'recipe' examples given throughout this book will give you direction on which oils to use and when. Have your dark-coloured bottle or jar standing by. You'll be adding the base oil or cream into the container just prior to the essential oils. A glass measuring beaker can be used to accurately deliver the right quantity of base oil.

The formula for mixing essential oils with a base oil or aromatherapy base cream (measured in grams as it is not easy to measure it in mls) is as follows:

As an adult measure for every 2ml of base oil, add 1 drop of essential oil.
For every 2g of base cream, add 1 drop of essential oil.

For example: To 50ml (1⅔ fl oz) of base oil add 25 drops of essential oils. If you have an uneven number as a base oil quantity, say 15ml (½ fl oz), giving a total of 7.5 drops of essential oils, just round the figure up or down to 8 or 6 drops.

Usually no more than three or four essential oils are mixed into a blend. Always consider an essential oil's blending factor (which gives a rough indication of blending, see below) and note (top, mid or base, see below) when mixing aromatherapy blends.

Blending Factor

The blending factor does not indicate the quantity of essential oil drops to be placed into a blend. It is only a guide to be either light- or heavy-handed with the oil when mixing. For example, lavender has a blending factor of 7 and is usually in a higher amount in a blend compared with an oil such as lemongrass, whose blending factor is 1.

Notes

Top notes
Have a small molecular structure and are more volatile than other notes; they will evaporate quickly from a blend. Most citrus essential oils are top notes.

Middle notes
Are less volatile than top notes, yet more volatile than base notes.

Base notes

Have the largest molecular structure and are therefore the heaviest and least volatile of all essential oils. They will stay in a blend the longest.

It is said that a good aromatherapy blend contains a top, middle and base note. While this is desirable, it's not always easy to achieve. For instance, all the aphrodisiac essential oils — rose, ylang-ylang, sandalwood and so on — are base notes. There are various suggestions for this mix within the chapters of this book.

It is important to keep the lid on your essential oil bottle as much as possible. Replace the cap immediately after use. If you don't do this, the more volatile top notes can easily escape from the bottle, reducing the life of the oil.

Blending summary

➤ Refer to the note and blending factor of an essential oil.
➤ For every 2ml of base oil (or 2g of cream), add 1 drop of essential oil.
➤ Blending factors are a guide only to the amount of essential oil that is to be placed in a blend.
➤ Notes indicate the volatility and 'weight' of an essential oil; top notes are very volatile and are light, base notes are less volatile and heavy (they'll stay in a blend longer than top or middle notes).

THIRTY ESSENTIAL OILS

Around 30 essential oils are listed below. For convenience, they have been sorted into 'Energising/Stimulating' or 'Relaxing/Calming'. If an oil has both properties ie stimulating to the digestive area but acts as a strong sedative, the oil has been placed where the dominant property lies. As you go through the oils, start thinking about blends that you can make yourself. Always read the 'Safety' section before using the oils in a blend. Look in the Further Reading section for more information on oils not listed.

ENERGISING/STIMULATING

Basil*	Eucalyptus	Fennel	Geranium*
Juniper	Lemon	Lemon grass	Myrrh
Peppermint	Pine	Rosemary	Sage
Tea-tree	Thyme		

*These oils can also be calming or relaxing.

BASIL

Ocimum basilicum
'I have a clear head and feel good'
BLENDING FACTOR: 1
NOTE: Top
PARTS USED: Flowers and leaves are steam distilled.
ORIGIN: Africa, Asia, Europe (particularly France).
ACTIONS: Antidepressant, antiseptic, antispasmodic, carminative, digestive, assists menstruation, expectorant, reduces fever, increases milk secretion, nerve tonic, adrenal cortex stimulant (helping with stress).
MIND AND EMOTIONS: Relieves poor concentration, mild depression, stress, indecision, mental fatigue and boredom.
BODY: Insect repellent. Use for indigestion, poor appetite, bronchitis, coughs, earache, muscular spasms, migraine and lack of or scanty menstruation.
BUYING TIPS: Purchase French or sweet basil (*O. Basilicum* var. *album*) rather than Exotic basil (*O. basilicum* var. *basilicum*) which is more irritant.
BLENDS WELL WITH: Bergamot, clary sage, geranium, lemon, rosemary.

SAFETY: Use in small quantities only. Avoid during pregnancy.

Eucalyptus

Eucalyptus globulus and other species
'I can breathe!'
BLENDING FACTOR: 1
NOTE: Top
PARTS USED: Leaves and young twigs are steam distilled.
ORIGIN: Native to Australia. Cultivated in Australia, Spain, Portugal, Brazil, California, Russia and China.
ACTIONS: Analgesic, antirheumatic, strong antiseptic, antispasmodic, antiviral, antiparasitic, decongestant, expectorant, deodorant, detoxifier, diuretic, expels intestinal worms, heals wounds, lowers blood-sugar levels, warms and reddens skin, reduces fever, stimulant.
MIND AND EMOTIONS: Clears the mind, refreshing.
BODY: Insect repellent. Use for arthritis, asthma, chickenpox, catarrh, colds and flu, coughs, cystitis, fever, measles, malaria, poor circulation, rheumatism, sinusitis, worms, wounds.
BUYING TIPS: Blue gum eucalyptus is most commonly sold, although you'd buy the lemon-scented eucalyptus if a strong anti-fungal agent was required.
BLENDS WELL WITH: Cedarwood, lavender, lemon, marjoram, thyme, rosemary.
SAFETY: Non-irritant to skin when diluted.

Fennel

Foeniculum vulgare
'My milk is now flowing'
BLENDING FACTOR: 6 or less
NOTE: Middle-base
PARTS USED: Crushed seeds are steam distilled.

ORIGIN: Native to the Mediterranean. Hungary, Bulgaria, Germany, France, Italy and India produce the oil.
ACTIONS: Anti-inflammatory, antimicrobial, antiseptic, antispasmodic, carminative, circulatory stimulant, digestive, diuretic, induces menstruation, expectorant, induces lactation, laxative, assists spleen health, expels worms.
MIND AND EMOTIONS: Revitalising, balancing and restorative.
BODY: Use for anorexia, asthma, bronchitis, colic, constipation, flatulence, gout, insufficient milk, kidney stones, lack of menstruation, oedema, obesity, menopause, rheumatism.
BUYING TIPS: Purchase only sweet fennel for aromatherapy usage.
BLENDS WELL WITH: Geranium, lavender, rose, sandalwood.
SAFETY: Use in moderation. Bitter fennel (*F. vulgare* var. *amara*) should not be used on the skin. Sweet fennel (*F. vulgare* var. *dulce*) can be. Neither oil is to be used in epilepsy or during pregnancy.

Did You Know?
Fennel is used widely in confectionary because of its aniseed flavour.

Geranium

Pelargonium graveolens
'She seemed more grounded'
BLENDING FACTOR: 3
NOTE: Middle
PARTS USED: Leaves, stems and flowers are steam distilled.
ORIGIN: Native to South Africa. Reunion (formerly Bourbon) Island, Egypt, Russia and China produce the oil.
ACTIONS: Antidepressant, anti-inflammatory, antiseptic, astringent, diuretic, expels worms, antifungal, prevents bleeding or haemorrhage, adrenal cortex stimulant, heals wounds.

MIND AND EMOTIONS: Balances the mind and body, uplifting; relieves anxiety, depression and stress.
BODY: Mosquito repellent. Use for bruises, broken capillaries, eczema, oedema, poor circulation, premenstrual syndrome, menopause, nervous exhaustion, sore throat, lice, ringworm.
BUYING TIPS: Geranium is sometimes referred to as 'rose geranium' because it has a rose-like aroma. Check when purchasing another oil called 'Rose Geranium' which is a mixture of rose and geranium, instead of pure geranium oil.
BLENDS WELL WITH: Lavender, patchouli, rose, sandalwood.
SAFETY: Can produce contact dermatitis in highly sensitive people.

JUNIPER

Juniperus communis
'Cystitis isn't a problem any more'
BLENDING FACTOR: 4
NOTE: Middle
PARTS USED: The berries are steam distilled.
ORIGIN: Native to the northern hemisphere. Italy, France, Austria, The Czech Republic, Spain, Germany and Canada produce the oil.
ACTIONS: Antirheumatic, antiseptic, antiparasitic, antispasmodic, aphrodisiac, astringent, carminative, digestive tonic, detoxifier, diuretic, promotes menstruation, reddens the skin, nerve tonic, sedative, heals wounds.
MIND AND EMOTIONS: Cleansing and purifying (when draining people are near), protective, restoring and revitalising; relieves stress.
BODY: Use for acne, cystitis, dermatitis, eczema, flabby skin, fluid retention, haemorrhoids, gout, rheumatism, lack of or painful menstruation, nervous tension.
BUYING TIPS: Check that the juniper oil is derived from direct

steam distillation of the berries. There is an inferior oil available that is produced from fermented berries, a by-product of gin production.
BLENDS WELL WITH: Citrus oils, cedarwood, cypress, clary sage, geranium, pine, lavender, rosemary.
SAFETY: Avoid during pregnancy. Do not use in kidney disease. May be slightly irritating; use in moderation.

LEMON

Citrus limonum
'It's refreshing'
BLENDING FACTOR: 3
NOTE: Top
PART USED: The rind is expressed.
ORIGIN: Native to Asia. Italy, Cyprus, Guinea, Israel, South and North America produce the oil.
ACTIONS: Antimicrobial, antibacterial, antirheumatic, antiseptic, antispasmodic, astringent, carminative, promotes sweating, diuretic, prevents anaemia, reduces fever, stops bleeding, lowers blood pressure, expels worms.
MIND AND EMOTIONS: Mental stimulant, refreshing, reviving.
BODY: Use for acne, arthritis, asthma, brittle nails, catarrh, corns, herpes, high blood pressure, poor circulation, obesity, rheumatism, nose bleeds, varicose veins, worms.
BUYING TIPS: Lemon oil can sometimes be tampered with to remove or reduce the terpene (a constituent of lemon oil) content. This increases the oil's irritability to the skin. For aromatherapy, the pure oil is essential.
BLENDS WELL WITH: Citrus oils, chamomile, eucalyptus, fennel, geranium, lavender, rose, ylang-ylang.
SAFETY: Phototoxic ... do not use on skin that will be exposed to direct sunlight. May cause skin irritations.

Lemongrass

Cymbopogon citratus
'My acne's gone!'
BLENDING FACTOR: 1
NOTE: Top
PARTS USED: The leaves are steam distilled.
ORIGIN: There are two species: one is native to the west of India, and is produced in Guatemala and India; the other is native to the east of India, and is produced in India.
ACTIONS: Analgesic, antidepressant, highly antimicrobial, antiseptic and antibacterial, antifungal, carminative, reduces fever, nerve tonic, sedative.
MIND AND EMOTIONS: Energising, refreshing, purifies the emotions; relieves anxiety and stress.
BODY: Insect repellent. Use for acne, fever, digestive disorders, headaches, infectious diseases, muscle pain, nervous exhaustion, flabby tissue.
BUYING TIPS: Take care to buy true lemongrass because it is sometimes referred to as 'citronella' (the famous insect repellent). Citronella is actually another species (*Cymbopogon nardus*).
BLENDS WELL WITH: Basil, eucalyptus, tea-tree, rosemary.
SAFETY: Use in moderation; may cause skin irritation in sensitive people.

Myrrh

Commiphora myrrha
'I feel restored'
BLENDING FACTOR: 7 or less
NOTE: Base
PART USED: The resin is extracted by solvent.
ORIGIN: Native to north-eastern Africa and south-western Asia.
ACTIONS: Antifungal, anti-inflammatory, antimicrobial, antiseptic, astringent, reduces catarrh, carminative, digestive,

induces menstruation, expectorant, sedative, uterus tonic, heals wounds.
MIND AND EMOTION: Revitalising, uplifting, restorative, soothing.
BODY: Use for arthritis, asthma, athlete's foot, bronchitis, catarrh, coughs, diarrhoea, digestive problems, eczema, lack of menstruation, ringworm, thrush.
BUYING TIPS: A 'sticky' myrrh oil is a sign of a poor quality oil.
BLENDS WELL WITH: Cypress, frankincense, geranium, lavender, peppermint, pine, sandalwood.
SAFETY: Use in moderation. Do not use in pregnancy.

Peppermint

Mentha piperita
'His tummy felt better'
BLENDING FACTOR: 3
NOTE: Middle
PART USED: The whole plant is steam distilled.
ORIGIN: Native to Europe. The oil is produced in Australia among other countries.
ACTIONS: Analgesic, anti-inflammatory, antiseptic, antispasmodic, astringent, digestive, expectorant, expels worms, induces menstruation, induces sweating, reduces fever, mind stimulant.
MIND AND EMOTION: Clears the mind, promotes positive thoughts, refreshing.
BODY: Use for colic, diarrhoea, flatulence, indigestion, nausea, vomiting, asthma, bronchitis, colds, coughs, sinusitis, rheumatism.
BUYING TIPS: A colourless oil (often found in supermarkets) indicates a modified oil. Use peppermint oil with a hint of colour for aromatherapy. As a general rule, most authentic essential oil should have 'colour'.

BLENDS WELL WITH: Eucalyptus, lavender, lemon, marjoram, rosemary.
SAFETY: Use in moderation. Avoid use in pregnancy.

PINE

Pinus sylvestris
'The infection cleared quickly'
BLENDING FACTOR: 3
NOTE: Middle
PARTS USED: Needles are dry distilled. Pine is used to produce turpentine.
ORIGIN: Native to Eurasia, and cultivated in the east of the United States, Europe, Russia, the Baltic states and Scandinavia.
ACTIONS: Highly antimicrobial, antibacterial and antiseptic, reduces nerve pain, antirheumatic, expectorant, expels worms, induces bile secretion, adrenal cortex and circulatory and nervous system stimulant.
MIND AND EMOTIONS: Mental stimulant, restorative, refreshing; relieves stress.
BODY: Use for arthritis, asthma, bronchitis, catarrh, coughs, colds and flu, cystitis, fatigue, gout, muscle aches, poor circulation, nervous exhaustion, nerve pain.
BUYING TIPS: Use only 'pure' pine oil for aromatherapy.
BLENDS WELL WITH: Cedarwood, eucalyptus, juniper, lavender, lemon, marjoram, rosemary, tea-tree.
SAFETY: Avoid use with allergic or sensitive individuals.

ROSEMARY

Rosmarinus officinalis
'My memory improved'
BLENDING FACTOR: 2
NOTE: Middle
PARTS USED: Flowers and leaves are steam distilled.
ORIGIN: Native to the Mediterranean. It is grown worldwide,

but the oil is produced mainly in France, Spain (poorer quality) and Tunisia.

ACTIONS: Adrenal cortex, circulatory system, liver and gall bladder stimulant, analgesic, antimicrobial, highly antiseptic, antirheumatic, induces bile secretion, carminative, digestive, diuretic, induces menstruation, mental stimulant, induces sweating, liver and nerve tonic, raises blood pressure, anti-sebaceous.

MIND AND EMOTIONS: Clarifies thinking, improves concentration, revitalising.

BODY: Insect repellent. Use for arthritis, aches and pains, asthma, bronchitis, diarrhoea, gout, jaundice, gall stones, headaches, painful menstruation, flatulence, rheumatism, poor circulation.

BUYING TIPS: Do not buy the Spanish rosemary oil that is produced from the whole plant. It is not used in aromatherapy.

BLENDS WELL WITH: Basil, cedarwood, lavender, peppermint, petitgrain, pine, thyme.

SAFETY: Not to be used in pregnancy or epilepsy or high blood pressure.

Did You Know?

You can make a quick 'pick-me-up' drink by placing a sprig of rosemary in a cup of boiling water. Let it stand for a few minutes and drink up.

SAGE

Salvia officinalis
'The flushes stopped'
BLENDING FACTOR: 4 or less
NOTE: Middle
PARTS USED: Dried leaves are steam distilled.
ORIGIN: Native to southern Europe, and cultivated worldwide.

ACTIONS: Antimicrobial, antiseptic, antispasmodic, astringent, digestive, diuretic, induces menstruation, laxative, raises blood pressure, reduces fever.
MIND AND EMOTIONS: Stimulating, refreshing.
BODY: Use for asthma, bacterial infections, lack of menstruation, menopause.
BUYING TIPS: Some aromatherapists prefer to use clary sage instead of common sage for therapeutic use.
BLENDS WELL WITH: Citrus oils, lavender, rosemary.
SAFETY: Use with extreme care and in moderation. Potentially toxic if applied directly to the skin. Avoid in pregnancy and epilepsy and high blood pressure.

Tea-tree

Melaleuca alternifolia
'The thrush went quickly'
BLENDING FACTOR: 3
NOTE: Top
PARTS USED: Leaves and twigs are steam distilled.
ORIGIN: Native to and produced in Australia.
ACTIONS: Highly antibacterial, antiviral, antiseptic and antifungal, anti-inflammatory, expectorant, immune system stimulant, induces sweating.
MIND AND EMOTIONS: Clears confusion, refreshing, purifies thoughts.
BODY: Use for acne, asthma, athlete's foot, bronchitis, catarrh, coughs, sinusitis, whooping cough, cold sores, colds and flu, fever, infectious disease, thrush, vaginitis.
BUYING TIPS: To avoid confusion all the *Melaleuca* family trees are referred to as tea-trees. *M. alternifolia* is the most common species used in aromatherapy.
BLENDS WELL WITH: Clary sage, geranium, lavender, lemon, marjoram, pine, rosemary.
SAFETY: Some people may be sensitive to it.

Thyme

Thymus vulgaris
'No more blackheads!'
BLENDING FACTOR: 1-2
NOTE: Middle
PARTS USED: Leaves and flowers are steam distilled.
ORIGIN: Native to Spain and southern Europe. The oil is produced mainly in Spain.
ACTIONS: Highly antibacterial, antifungal, antiseptic, antivenom and antimicrobial, antirheumatic, antispasmodic, astringent, aphrodisiac, eases coughing, diuretic, expectorant, expels intestinal worms, general stimulant, induces menstruation, nerve tonic, raises blood pressure.
MIND AND EMOTIONS: Mentally stimulating, purifies thoughts, restorative.
BODY: Use for acne, asthma, arthritis, bronchitis, catarrh, coughs, colds and flu, diarrhoea, gout, headache, poor circulation, rheumatism, sinusitis, tonsillitis.
BUYING TIPS: There are six different essential oils that are produced from *T. vulgaris*. No one quite knows why. The 'sweet' thyme oils are used by lay aromatherapists. Whereas the 'red' thyme oils should only be used by a practitioner.
BLENDS WELL WITH: Bergamot, lavender, lemon, marjoram, pine.
SAFETY: Use with care and in moderation; can cause skin irritation in some people. Do not use in pregnancy or with high blood pressure.

Relaxing/Calming

Bergamot	Cedarwood	Chamomile	Clary sage
Cypress	Frankincense	Lavender	Marjoram
Neroli	Orange	Patchouli	Petitgrain
Rose	Sandalwood	Vetiver	Ylang-ylang

BERGAMOT

Citrus bergamia
'Keeps me calm and positive'
BLENDING FACTOR: 10
NOTE: Top-Middle
PART USED: Rind of ripe fruit is expressed.
ORIGIN: Asia and Italy (main source).
ACTIONS: Analgesic, antidepressant (uplifting and calming), urinary and pulmonary antiseptic, antispasmodic, carminative, deodorant, digestive, diuretic, expels intestinal worms, general stimulant, reduces fever, heals wounds, reddens skin.
MIND AND EMOTIONS: Relieves anxiety, depression, fear, nightmares and stress; promotes positive thoughts.
BODY: Insect repellent. Use for acne, boils, cold sores, cystitis, eczema, dermatitis, eating disorders (anorexia), flatulence, thrush, worms, wounds.
BUYING TIPS: Take care not to confuse the other 'bergamot' (*monardo didyma*) for *citrus bergamia*. Begamot is responsible for the 'Earl Grey' tea flavour, have a look in the supermarket.
BLENDS WELL WITH: Chamomile, cypress, geranium, juniper, lavender, lemon.
SAFETY: Phototoxic, can cause skin pigmentation and sensitisation when exposed to direct sunlight. If in doubt, ask your aromatherapist for advice.

CEDARWOOD

Juniperus virginiana
'I feel so much better'
BLENDING FACTOR: 4
NOTE: Base
PARTS USED: Timber sawdust and shavings are steam distilled.
ORIGIN: Native to North America.
ACTIONS: Antispasmodic, astringent, diuretic, expectorant, induces menstruation, increases circulation, reduces oil

secretions (sweat glands), sedative, urinary and pulmonary antiseptic.

MIND AND EMOTIONS: Soothes, calms, relieves anxiety, releases mental tension.

BODY: Use for acne, arthritis, bronchitis, catarrh, cystitis, cough, eczema, nervous tension, psoriasis, rheumatism, sinusitis.

BUYING TIPS: Most pencils are made of cedarwood. The off-cuts from this make the commonly available oil. A more superior (and expensive) oil comes from the heartwood.

BLENDS WELL WITH: Clary sage, bergamot, geranium, lavender, lemon, marjoram, neroli, patchouli, rose.

SAFETY: Abortive, not to be used in pregnancy. May cause skin irritation to sensitive individuals.

CHAMOMILE

Matricaria chamomilla (German chamomile)
Anthemis nobilis (Roman chamomile)
'My angry skin calmed down'
BLENDING FACTOR: 1
NOTE: Middle
PARTS USED: Flower heads are steam distilled.
ORIGIN: Native to Europe and Asia. The oil is produced in Hungary and eastern Europe.
ACTIONS: Analgesic, anti-allergic (German more so), antispasmodic, antibacterial, antifungal, carminative, digestive, expels intestinal worms, heals wounds, increases white blood cell production, induces sweating, induces menstruation, liver and spleen tonic, sedative, reduces fever, reduces inflammation.
MIND AND EMOTIONS: Comforts and calms; relieves anxiety, hysteria, fretting, irritability and stress.
BODY: Use for acne, allergies, arthritis, colic, dermatitis, eczema, headaches, indigestion, insect bites, insomnia, migraine, painful or excessive bleeding during menstruation, menopause, rashes, rheumatism, toothache.

BUYING TIPS: Chamomile teabags (squeezed) can help to relieve conjunctivitis when placed on the eyes.
BLENDS WELL WITH: Bergamot, cypress, lavender, lemon, marjoram, rose.
SAFETY: Can cause dermatitis in a few individuals.

Clary Sage

Salvia sclarea
'Let's party'
BLENDING FACTOR: 4
NOTE: Middle–Base
PARTS USED: Flowers and leaves are steam distilled.
ORIGIN: Native to Europe, and cultivated worldwide.
ACTIONS: Antidepressant, antiseptic, antibacterial, antispasmodic, anti-sebaceous, aphrodisiac, astringent, carminative, deodorant, digestive, induces menstruation, lowers blood pressure, nerve tonic and sedative, prevents convulsions, uterus tonic.
MIND AND EMOTIONS: Balancing, inspiring, relaxing, euphoric and revitalising; relieves fear, irritability, depression and drained feelings.
BODY: Use for aches and pains, acne, asthma, colic, dandruff, high blood pressure, migraine, lack of or painful menstruation.
BUYING TIPS: Take care not to confuse the oil with the more irritant 'sage' oil.
BLENDS WELL WITH: Cedarwood, citrus oils, frankincense, geranium, juniper, marjoram, lavender, pine, sandalwood.
SAFETY: Do not use in pregnancy. Do not use clary sage while drinking alcohol as it will exaggerate drunkenness.

Cypress

Cupressus sempervirens
'I don't sweat as much any more'

BLENDING FACTOR: 5
NOTE: Middle
PARTS USED: Needles and twigs are steam distilled.
ORIGIN: Native to southern Europe and western Asia. The oil is produced in France, Spain and Morocco.
ACTIONS: Antirheumatic, antiseptic, antispasmodic, astringent, constricts blood vessels, deodorant, diuretic, liver tonic, reduces sweating, stops bleeding.
MIND AND EMOTIONS: Purifying, soothing, restorative, reviving and warming; relieves anxiety, low spirits, uncontrolled crying, stress and irritability.
BODY: Insect repellent. Use for asthma, bronchitis, excessive sweating, haemorrhoids, muscular cramps, oedema, painful or excessive menstruation, menopause, varicose veins.
BUYING TIPS: If you have high blood pressure check to see which part of the plant has been used to make the oil before purchasing.
BLENDS WELL WITH: Cedarwood, citrus oils, chamomile, clary sage, juniper, majoram, lavender, pine, sandalwood.
SAFETY: Oil from the cone should be avoided by high blood pressure sufferers.

Frankincense

Boswellia carteri
'It made meditation easier'
BLENDING FACTOR: 3
NOTE: Base
PART USED: Oleo gum resin is steam distilled.
ORIGIN: Native to Africa, Arabia and India. The oil is produced in Europe and India.
ACTIONS: Antiseptic, astringent, carminative, digestive, diuretic, expectorant, induces menstruation, anti-inflammatory, sedative, uterus tonic, heals wounds.
MIND AND EMOTIONS: Clears the mind, protective, purifying

and uplifting; relieves anxiety, nervous tension, depression and stress; assists meditation, yoga and prayer.
BODY: Use for asthma, bronchitis, catarrh, colds and flu, coughs, cystitis, painful menstruation.
BUYING TIPS: As a guide the 'real thing' is usually four times more expensive than orange oil.
BLENDS WELL WITH: Basil, bergamot, geranium, lavender, neroli, pine, sandalwood, vetiver.
SAFETY: Nil.

LAVENDER

Lavandula angustifolia, L. officinalis, L. spica
'I use it almost every day!'
BLENDING FACTOR: 7
NOTE: Top - Middle
PARTS USED: Flowers are steam distilled.
ORIGIN: Native to the Mediterranean. The oil is produced in many regions, including in Tasmania (mainly *L. angustifolia*). *L. officinalis* is mainly produced in France.
ACTIONS: Analgesic, antidepressant, antimicrobial, antirheumatic, antiseptic, antispasmodic, carminative, deodorant, detoxifier, diuretic, expels intestinal worms, induces bile secretion, induces menstruation, insecticide, liver tonic, lowers blood pressure, nerve tonic, prevents convulsions, sedative, heals wounds. The most versatile essential oil!
MIND AND EMOTIONS: Balancing, calming, cleansing, purifying, relaxing, restorative and soothing; relieves anxiety, restlessness, depression, fear, overactive mind and hysteria.
BODY: Use for acne, allergies, asthma, bronchitis, burns, catarrh, cystitis, colic, dandruff, dermatitis, earache, eczema, flatulence, headaches, insomnia, lice, migraine, muscular aches, nausea, premenstrual tension, rheumatism, wounds.
BUYING TIPS: Take care not to confuse this with cheap lavandin oil (a cross between *L. angustifolia/officinalis* and spike lavender). Tasmanian lavender oil is one of the best.

BLENDS WELL WITH: Most oils.
SAFETY: Nil.

Marjoram

Origanum majorana
'I slept like a baby'
BLENDING FACTOR: 3
NOTE: Middle
PARTS USED: Flowers and leaves are steam distilled.
ORIGIN: Native to the Mediterranean, and cultivated worldwide.
ACTIONS: Analgesic, anti-oxidant, antiseptic, antispasmodic, antibacterial, antifungal, antiviral, carminative, dilates blood vessels, digestive, diuretic, expectorant, laxative, lowers blood pressure, nerve tonic, prevents aphrodisiac, sedative, heals wounds.
MIND AND EMOTIONS: Comforting, restorative and warming; relieves anxiety, lack of sleep, mental fatigue and stress.
BODY: Use for arthritis, asthma, bronchitis, colic, coughs, constipation, flatulence, headache, high blood pressure, insomnia, lack of or painful menstruation, muscular aches and pains, nervous tension, premenstrual tension.
BUYING TIPS: Ensure you are buying *O. marjorana* not a poor substitute called Spanish marjoram (*T. mastichina*).
BLENDS WELL WITH: Bergamot, cedarwood, chamomile, cypress, eucalyptus, lavender, tea-tree.
SAFETY: Do not use in pregnancy.

Neroli (Orange Blossom)

Citrus aurantium, var. *amara* (bitter), var. *Sinensis* (sweet)
'It's the key 'shock' remedy'
BLENDING FACTOR: 2
NOTE: Base
PARTS USED: Enfleurage is still used in some places. Flowers are also steam distilled to produce orange water.

ORIGIN: Native to the Far East, and cultivated in France, Tunisia, Italy and the United States.

ACTIONS: Antidepressant, antiseptic, antispasmodic, aphrodisiac, antibacterial, antifungal, carminative, digestive, deodorant, heart tonic, mild hypnotic, nerve stimulant.

MIND AND EMOTIONS: Hypnotic, restorative, soothing and uplifting; relieves anxiety, depression, grief, restlessness and shock.

BODY: Use for colic, diarrhoea, flatulence, nervous dyspepsia and tension, palpitations, premenstrual tension, poor circulation.

BUYING TIPS: As a guide, neroli is usually 30 times more expensive than orange oil. An affordable neroli can be bought diluted in base oil.

BLENDS WELL WITH: Most oils.

SAFETY: Nil.

Orange

Citrus aurantium, var. *amara* (bitter), var. *sinensis* (sweet)
'I don't feel down any more'
BLENDING FACTOR: 2 or more
NOTE: Top
PART USED: Rind is expressed.
ORIGIN: Native to China and India. Oil is produced in Israel, Cyprus, Brazil and North America.

ACTIONS: Antidepressant, antiseptic, antibacterial, antifungal, carminative, digestive, lowers blood pressure, increases bile flow, anti-inflammatory, sedative.

MIND AND EMOTIONS: Comforting, refreshing, soothing and uplifting; relieves anxiety, emotional exhaustion and stress.

BODY: Use for bronchitis, colds and flu, constipation, dyspepsia, insomnia.

BUYING TIPS: Bitter and sweet orange oil have similar properties. Sweet orange has a milder effect and would be the preferred choice in children's remedies.

BLENDS WELL WITH: Clary sage, lavender, lemon, myrrh, neroli, sandalwood.
SAFETY: Use in moderation. May cause skin irritation or rash when exposed to direct sunlight.

Patchouli

Pogostemon cablin
'The 'skin' essential oil'
BLENDING FACTOR: 5
NOTE: Base
PARTS USED: Leaves are steam distilled.
ORIGIN: Native to Asia. Oil is produced in India, Indonesia, China, the Philippines, Malaysia and South America.
ACTIONS: Antidepressant, antimicrobial, antibacterial, antiseptic, aphrodisiac, carminative, deodorant, digestive, diuretic, nerve tonic, anti-inflammatory, reduces nausea, vomiting and fever.
MIND AND EMOTIONS: Uplifting, calming and appeasing; relieves anxiety and stress.
BODY: Use as skin remedy for acne, eczema, dermatitis, cracked skin, and wound healing; use for frigidity and nervous exhaustion.
BUYING TIPS: Usually one of the more expensive oils.
BLENDS WELL WITH: Bergamot, cedarwood, clary sage, geranium, lavender, myrrh, neroli, rose, sandalwood, vetiver.
SAFETY: Nil.

Petitgrain

Citrus aurantium, var. *amara* (bitter)
'I feel good'
BLENDING FACTOR: 2
NOTE: Middle
PARTS USED: Leaves and twigs of the bitter orange tree are steam distilled.

ORIGIN: Native to China and India. It's the best oil produced in France.

ACTIONS: Antiseptic, antispasmodic, deodorant, digestive, nerve tonic, general tonic.

MIND AND EMOTIONS: Balancing, refreshing, revitalising and stimulates the mind; relieves anxiety and stress.

BODY: Use for acne, colic, convalescence, flatulence, indigestion.

BUYING TIPS: If you can't afford neroli, buy petitgrain — a poorer cousin.

BLENDS WELL WITH: Citrus oils, clary sage, geranium, lavender.

SAFETY: May cause skin reactions if exposed to direct sunlight.

ROSE

Rosa centifolia, R. damascena
'Love is in the air'
BLENDING FACTOR: 1
NOTE: Base
PARTS USED: Rose otto by steam distillation of fresh petals. Fresh petals by enfleurage to produce an absolute (very expensive).

ORIGIN: Oil is mainly produced in France, Morocco and Turkey.

ACTIONS: Antidepressant, antiseptic, antispasmodic, aphrodisiac, astringent, induces bile secretion, induces menstruation, anti-inflammatory, stops bleeding by coagulation, heart, stomach, liver, spleen and uterus tonic.

MIND AND EMOTIONS: Comforting, appeasing, soothing and uplifting; relieves; anger, depression, grief, jealousy, shock and emotional stress.

BODY: Use for asthma, coughs, nausea, palpitations, liver congestion, impotence, frigidity, sinusitis headaches, menstrual irregularities, poor circulation.

BUYING TIPS: Instead of the very expensive pure rose oil, you

can buy an affordable, diluted (with jojoba) rose oil to enjoy.
BLENDS WELL WITH: Bergamot, chamomile, clary sage, geranium, lavender, neroli, sandalwood.
SAFETY: Nil.

SANDALWOOD

Santalum album
'Peaceful and calm'
BLENDING FACTOR: 6 or less
NOTE: Base
PARTS USED: Roots and heartwood are steam distilled.
ORIGIN: Native to Asia. Mysore in India produces the best oil.
ACTIONS: Antidepressant, antispasmodic, aphrodisiac, astringent, antibacterial, antifungal, urinary and pulmonary antiseptic, diuretic, expectorant, insecticide, sedative, general tonic, reduces inflammation.
MIND AND EMOTIONS: Elevating, relaxing, uplifting, soothing and grounding; relieves stress, anxiety, depression, heartaches and sexual problems linked with anxiety.
BODY: Use for bronchitis, catarrh, cystitis, dry coughs, diarrhoea, nausea, insomnia, sore throat.
BUYING TIPS: Check the label. Don't get caught out paying Mysore (east Indian) prices for the inferior west of India or Australian oil.
BLENDS WELL WITH: Bergamot, lavender, myrrh, patchouli, rose, vetiver.
SAFETY: Nil.

VETIVER

Vetiveria zizanioides
'The oil of tranquillity'
BLENDING FACTOR: 1
NOTE: Base
PARTS USED: Roots are steam distilled.

ORIGIN: Native to India and Sri Lanka. Oil is produced in Java, Haiti, Europe and the United States.
ACTIONS: Antiseptic, antispasmodic, detoxifier, expels worms, increases circulation, strong sedative, tonic.
MIND AND EMOTIONS: Calming, grounding, mental sedative, soothing and uplifting; relieves anxiety, depression, insomnia, oversensitivity and scattered energy.
BODY: Arthritis, aches and pains, insomnia, nervous tension.
BUYING TIPS: As I've mentioned, this oil smells like a swamp, buy it anyway! It's the tranquility oil.
BLENDS WELL WITH: Frankincense, patchouli, sandalwood, ylang-ylang.
SAFETY: Nil.

YLANG-YLANG

Cananga odorata
'The aphrodisiac'
BLENDING FACTOR: 4
NOTE: Base
PARTS USED: Fresh flowers are steam distilled.
ORIGIN: Native to Asia. Oil producers include Madagascar, Europe, the Comoro Islands and United States.
ACTIONS: Antidepressant, antiseptic, aphrodisiac, euphoric, lowers blood pressure, nerve tonic, reduces oil secretion from sweat glands, sedative.
MIND AND EMOTIONS: Appeasing, calming, euphoric, soothing; relieves anxiety, depression, impatience, irritability, heartache, sexual problems of mental/emotional origin, and stress.
BODY: Use for frigidity, high blood pressure, impotence, insomnia, palpitations.
BUYING TIPS: There are many grades of ylang-ylang available to essential oil suppliers. Buying this oil from a reputable supplier will hopefully mean a more superior oil has been bottled.
BLENDS WELL WITH: Bergamot, rose, vetiver.
SAFETY: Use in moderation. May cause skin irritation in some

individuals. Care should be taken with people who suffer low blood pressure.

SUMMARY CHARTS

MIND AND EMOTIONS

Use the following oils in a:
- Massage
- Bath
- Aromatherapy burner
- Inhalation
- Tissue

ESSENTIAL OILS FOR POSITIVE CHANGE

State	Essential oil
Anger	Chamomile, rose, ylang-ylang
Anxiety	Bergamot, cedarwood, chamomile, geranium, lavender, marjoram, neroli, orange, patchouli, petitgrain, sandalwood
Confusion	Basil, cypress, peppermint, frankincense
Confidence	Frankincense
Depression	Bergamot, chamomile, clary sage, geranium, lavender, neroli, orange, patchouli, peppermint, rose, sandalwood
Fatigue	Basil, geranium, lemon, lemongrass, marjoram, peppermint pine, rosemary

Fear	Chamomile, clary sage
Frustration	Rose, ylang-ylang
Grief	Bergamot, marjoram, neroli, rose
Guilt	Cypress, marjoram, neroli, orange, petitgrain
Hysteria	Chamomile, clary sage, lavender, marjoram, neroli, peppermint, vetiver
Insomnia	Chamomile, lavender, marjoram, neroli, sandalwood, vetiver
Impatience	Bergamot, chamomile, clary sage, cypress, rose
Jealousy	Rose
Shock	Neroli

BODY

The following charts show aromatherapy solutions to the body's health problems. The essential oil, preferred usage and a chapter reference for an aromatherapy 'recipe' example are included for each section.

HEAD AND CHEST

PROBLEM	ESSENTIAL OIL	AROMATHERAPY USE	'RECIPE' EXAMPLE
Asthma	Benzoin, bergamot, clary sage, cypress, eucalyptus, frankincense, marjoram, peppermint, rose	Massage Steam inhalation Aromatherapy burner (Benzoin is a resin)	Ch. 3

Bronchitis	Basil, benzoin, cypress, eucalyptus, frankincense, lavender, myrrh, pine, rosemary, sandalwood, tea-tree	Chest and back massage Steam inhalation Aromatherapy burner	Ch. 3
Catarrh	Cedarwood, eucalyptus, frankincense, lavender, myrrh, peppermint, pine, rosemary, sandalwood, tea-tree, thyme	As above	Ch 3
Colds and flu	Basil, eucalyptus, lemon, lemongrass, marjoram, peppermint, rosemary, tea-tree	As above	Ch. 3
Coughs	Benzoin, cedarwood, eucalyptus, frankincense, marjoram, myrrh, peppermint, pine, sandalwood	As above	—
Earache	Chamomile, mullein, tea-tree	Warm compress	Ch. 3
Headache	Chamomile, eucalyptus, lavender, lemon grass, marjoram, peppermint, rosemary	Head, neck and shoulder massage Aromatherapy burner	Ch. 5

Laryngitis	Benzoin, frankincense, lavender, myrrh, sandalwood, thyme	Steam inhalation	—
Migraine	Chamomile, basil, lavender, peppermint	Compress Aromatherapy burner	Ch. 6
Sinusitis	Eucalyptus, peppermint, pine, tea-tree	Steam inhalation	Ch. 6
Teething	Chamomile	Warm compress on cheek	Ch. 3
Throat infection	Bergamot, clary sage, geranium, lavender, pine, sandalwood, tea-tree, thyme	Steam inhalation	Ch. 3 (see *tonsillitis*)
Tonsillitis	Bergamot, lavender, tea-tree, thyme, lemongrass	Gentle throat massage	Ch. 3

DIGESTIVE SYSTEM

PROBLEM	ESSENTIAL OIL	AROMATHERAPY USE	'RECIPE' EXAMPLE
Colic	Chamomile, lavender, marjoram, peppermint	Gentle abdominal massage	Ch. 3
Constipation	Fennel, marjoram, orange, lavender, rosemary	General or abdominal massage Hip bath or full bath	Ch. 4

Diarrhoea	Chamomile, cypress, fennel, geranium, peppermint, sandalwood	Abdominal massage Bath	Ch. 4 (see *constipation*)
Flatulence	Chamomile, fennel, lavender, marjoram, orange, peppermint	Abdominal massage	Ch. 4 (see *constipation*)
Heartburn/ Indigestion	Chamomile, clary sage, fennel, marjoram, orange, peppermint	Massage Aromatherapy burner	Ch. 5
Nausea/ Vomiting	Chamomile, fennel, lavender, peppermint	Tissue Aromatherapy burner	Chs. 5 and 6
Poor appetite	Bergamot, myrrh	Massage Aromatherapy burner	—

MUSCLES AND JOINTS

PROBLEM	ESSENTIAL OIL	AROMATHERAPY USE	'RECIPE' EXAMPLE
Arthritis/ Rheumatism	Chamomile, eucalyptus, juniper, lavender, marjoram, peppermint, pine, rosemary	Massage Bath Compress on area	Ch. 6
Cramp	Cypress, lavender, marjoram, rosemary	Massage area	Ch. 7
Gout	Benzoin, juniper, pine, rosemary	Gentle massage Foot bath or full bath	Ch. 6

Problem	Essential oil	Aromatherapy use	'Recipe' example
Poor muscle tone	Juniper, rosemary	Regular massage	Ch. 7
Sprains/Strains	Chamomile, lavender, marjoram, pine	Cold compress	Ch. 7

Urinary and reproductive tracts

Problem	Essential oil	Aromatherapy use	'Recipe' example
Absent menstruation	Clary sage, fennel, juniper, marjoram, myrrh, rose	Massage area Bath	Ch. 4
Cystitis	Bergamot, cedarwood, chamomile, juniper, lavender, pine, sandalwood, tea-tree	Douche Bath	Ch. 4
Frigidity	Neroli, patchouli, rose, sandalwood, ylang-ylang	Massage Aromatherapy burner	Ch. 5
Heavy menstruation	Chamomile, cypress, geranium, rose	Massage area Bath	Ch. 4
Impotence	Clary sage, rose, sandalwood, ylang-ylang	Body massage Bath	Ch. 6
Menopause	Cypress, fennel, geranium, rose	Massage Bath Aromatherapy burner	Ch. 5

Painful or irregular menstruation	Basil, chamomile, clary sage, cypress, frankincense, juniper, lavender, marjoram, rose	Massage Bath Warm compress Aromatherapy burner	Ch. 4
Premenstrual syndrome	Chamomile, geranium, lavender, marjoram, neroli	Massage Bath Aromatherapy burner	Ch. 4
Thrush	Bergamot, myrrh, tea-tree	Bath Douche	Ch. 5
Urethritis	Bergamot, lavender, tea-tree	Bath Douche	Ch. 4 (see cystitis)
Vaginal itching	Bergamot, cedarwood, frankincense, lavender, myrrh, sandalwood, tea-tree	Bath Douche	Ch. 5

SKIN AND CIRCULATORY SYSTEM

PROBLEM	ESSENTIAL OIL	AROMATHERAPY USE	'RECIPE' EXAMPLE
Athlete's foot	Lavender, lemongrass, myrrh, patchouli, tea-tree	Powder	Ch. 6
Bites/Stings	Chamomile, lavender, tea-tree	Swab	Chs. 3 and 6
Boils	Bergamot, chamomile, lavender, lemon, tea-tree, thyme	Swab Bath	Ch. 1

Bruises	Lavender (Also homoeopathic Arnica)	Compress Swab	Chs. 3 and 7
Burns	Lavender, tea-tree	Neat Lavender Gentle massage	Chs. 3 and 6
Cuts/Sores	Lavender, tea-tree	Compress Gentle massage	Ch. 3
Dermatitis	Cedarwood, chamomile, geranium, juniper, lavender, neroli, rose, thyme	Massage Bath Compress	Ch. 4
Eczema	Bergamot, cedarwood, chamomile, geranium, juniper, lavender, myrrh, patchouli, rose, thyme	Massage Bath Compress	Ch. 4
Fluid retention	Cypress, fennel, geranium, juniper, orange, rosemary	Massage Bath	Ch. 4
Haemorrhoids	Cypress, juniper, myrrh	Gentle massage Bath	Ch. 5
Herpes	Bergamot, tea-tree	Swab Douche (genital)	Ch. 4
High blood pressure	Lavender, lemon, marjoram, clary sage, ylang-ylang	Massage Bath Aromatherapy burner	Ch. 6
Low blood pressure	Juniper, peppermint, rosemary, thyme	Massage Bath Aromatherapy burner	Ch. 5

Obesity	Fennel, juniper, lemon, orange	Massage Bath	Ch. 4
Palpitations	Orange, neroli, rose, ylang-ylang	Massage	Ch. 6
Poor circulation	Cypress, eucalyptus, geranium, neroli, pine, rose, rosemary, thyme	Massage Bath	Chs. 6 and 8
Varicose veins	Cypress, lemon, neroli, rosemary	Compress	Ch. 5

SAFETY INFORMATION

When used correctly, essential oils can have positive and therapeutic effects on the mind, body and emotions. They are not recommended for internal use and it is important to read and follow the 'Safety' section of each essential oil's description. The information below pertains to the 30 essential oils covered in this chapter. For information on essential oils not mentioned, please see the Further Reading section.

Alcohol: Clary sage increases the effect of alcohol. Do not drink alcohol and use this essential oil.

Babies and children: Use essential oils according to the following guidelines:
Babies (to one year) Dilute 1 drop of lavender, chamomile, rose, tangerine in 10ml of base oil for massage or bath.
Infants (up to five years) Dilute 2 drops of safe (chamomile, lavender, cypress, geranium, lavender, rose, sandalwood, tea-tree, eucalyptus) non-irritant essential oils in 5–10ml of base oil for massage or bath.
Children (6–12 years) Dilute half the adult dose* of essential oils in base oil or bath; for example, 3 drops of essential oil in 10ml of base oil or 5 drops in 20ml (⅔ fl oz) of base oil.

Adults* (over 12 years) For every 2ml of base oil, add 1 drop of essential oil.

Epilepsy: These oils must be avoided by epileptics: fennel, rosemary, sage.

High blood pressure: Do not use the following oils in cases of high blood pressure, as they increase blood pressure: rosemary, sage, thyme.

Kidneys: Juniper should not be used on any person with kidney problems.

Phototoxic: Do not use these essential oils and go out into direct sunlight: bergamot, lemon, tangerine, orange and other citrus oils.

Pregnancy: The following oils are not to be used at all during pregnancy: basil, cedarwood, clary sage, fennel, juniper, marjoram, myrrh, peppermint, rosemary, sage, thyme. It is always best to consult an aromatherapist at this time.

Skin: A patch test is advisable for the oils mentioned below or any other oil you may be sensitive to. Place a diluted drop of the essential oil onto the back of your wrist. If it does not react within 12 hours it is safe to use. These oils may cause skin irritations: cedarwood, geranium, lemongrass, peppermint, pine, thyme.

Glossary

Analgesic a substance that reduces or deadens pain.
Anti-allergic a substance that combats an allergic reaction.
Antibacterial a substance that destroys certain bacteria.
Antidepressant a substance that helps to alleviate depression.
Antifungal a substance that destroys fungi.
Anti-inflammatory a substance that alleviates inflammation.
Antimicrobial a substance that destroys harmful micro-organisms.
Anti-oxidant a substance that reduces the deterioration or oxidation of certain materials.
Antiparasitic a substance that destroys parasites.
Antirheumatic a substance that helps to alleviate rheumatism.
Antisebaceous a substance which reduces the flow of sebum from the sebaceous gland.
Antispasmodic a substance that relieves spasm in smooth muscle.
Antiviral a substance that is effective against illness-causing viruses.
Aphrodisiac a substance that stimulates sexual arousal.
Astringent a substance that contracts or shrinks the tissues.
Carminative a substance that relieves flatulence.
Decongestant a substance that reduces congestion, usually of the mucous membranes.
Deodorant a substance that eliminates or masks foul odours.
Detoxifier a substance that eliminates toxins.
Digestive a substance that promotes the process of digestion.
Diuretic a substance that increases the elimination of urine.
Euphoric a substance that produces elated sensations.

Expectorant a substance that increases the elimination of catarrh from the chest area.
Hypnotic a substance which may cause sleep.
Insecticide a substance that destroys insects.
Laxative a substance that increases the frequency of elimination from the bowels.
Sedative a substance that has a calming effect.
Stimulant a substance that increases activity in a function or body system.
Tonic a substance that promotes well-being in the whole, or in specific parts, of the body.

FURTHER READING

The A–Z of First Aid and Family Health, Blitz Editions, Leicester UK, 1994.

Arcier, M. Aromatherapy Training Course, self-published notes.

Avery, A. *Aromatherapy and You: A Guide to Natural Skin Care*, Blue Heron Hill Press, Portland, Oregon, 1992.

Barraclough, D. *A Flower-Lover's Miscellany*, Frederick Warne & Co., London, 1961.

Basset, I. B. et al. 'A Comparative Study of Tea-tree Oil Versus Benzoylperoxide in the Treatment of Acne', *Medical Journal of Australia*, vol. 153, 1990, pp. 455–58.

Douglas, J. *The Australian Book of Aromatherapy*, Hale & Iremonger, Sydney, 1994.

Fletcher, K. *Essential Oils: Enhance Your Home and Workplace with the Natural Essence of Plants*, Penguin Books, Ringwood VIC, 1995.

Gattefossé, R. *Gattefosse's Aromatherapy*, The C. W. Daniel Company, Essex UK, 1993.

Harris, T. A. *I'm OK, You're OK*, Pan Books, London, 1970.

International Journal of Aromatherapy, Aromatherapy publications, Sussex UK.

Jackson, J. *Aromatherapy*, Dorling Kindersley, London, 1992.

Kennett, F. *History of Perfume*, Harrap, London, 1975.

Launert, E. *Scent and Scent Bottles*, Barrie & Jenkins, London, 1974.

Lawless, J. *Aromatherapy and the Mind: An Exploration into the Psychological and Emotional Effects of Essential Oils*, Thorsons, London, 1994.

Lawless, J. *The Encyclopaedia of Essential Oils*, Element, Rockport, 1992.

McGilvery, C. & Reed, J. *Essential Aromatherapy*, Anness Publishing, London, 1993.

Mowrey, D. B. *The Scientific Validation of Herbal Medicine*, Keats Publishing, New Canaan CT, 1986.

Oxford Reference: *Concise Medical Dictionary*, Oxford University Press, London, 1994.

Price, S. *Aromatherapy Workbook: Understanding Essential Oils from Plant to Bottle*, Thorsons, London, 1993.

Price, S. *Practical Aromatherapy: How to Use Essential Oils to Restore Vitality*, Thorsons, London, 1987.

Purchon, N. *Aromatherapy*, Hodder & Stoughton, Sydney, 1994.

Seymour-Apps, A. & Taylor, P. *The Aromatherapy Centre, Post-Graduate Coursebook*, 1992.

Tisserand, M. *Aromatherapy for Women*, Thorsons, London, 1990.

Tong et al. 'Tea-tree Oil in the Treatment of Tinea Pedis', *Australian Journal of Dermatology*, vol. 33, 1992, pp. 145–49.

Trueman, J. *The Romantic Story of Scent*, Aldus Books, London, 1975.

Van Troller, S. & Dodd, G. H. (eds). *Perfumery: The Psychology and Biology of Fragrance*, Chapmand & Hall, London, 1991.

Westcott, P. *Alternative Health Care for Women*, Collins, Sydney, 1987.

White, J. & Day, K. *Aromatherapy for Scentual Awareness*, Nacson & Sons, Sydney, 1993.

INDEX

A

abrasions, 41, 95
acne, 58–62
adolescents, 52–71
adulterated oils, 10–11
adventure sport, 112
ageing skin, 127
ailments, 168–175
    babies, 37–40
    children, 41–47
    men, 98
    teenagers, 58–69
    women, 79
allergies, skin, 126
anger, 56, 79, 97, 167
antibacterial oils, 126
anti-inflammatory oils, 126
anti-oxidant oils, 127
antisebaceous oils, 127
antiseptic oils, 127
anxiety, 35, 77, 121–122, 167
appetite, 171
apple masque, 134
aromatherapist
    choosing, 28–29
    training, 27–29
arthritis, 98–99, 171
asthma, 41, 168
astringent oils, 127
athlete's foot, 99–100, 173

B

back massage, 104
bacteria, skin, 126
balding, 110
base notes, 144
base or carrier oils, 20
basil, 145
baths, 15–16, 34, 85
beauty products, 124–140
bed-wetting, 41
bee sting, 41–42
bergamot, 156
bites, 173
blackheads, 132
blending essential oils, 142–144
blind children, 47–48

blood pressure, 82, 101, 174
body massage, 18
boils, 173
botanical names, 11
bottle colour, 12–13
bronchitis, 42, 169
bruises, 42, 113, 174
burner, 14–15, 35
burns, 42–43, 94, 174
buying essential oils, 10–13

C

calm, 55, 155–165
car, 93
carriers, 13–22
catarrh, 44, 95, 169
cedarwood, 156–157
cell regeneration, 127
chamomile, 130, 157–158
chest, 168–170
chickenpox, 44–45
childbirth, 89–91
circulation, 18, 127, 173–175
clary sage, 158
clay masques, 133–134
cleansing the skin, 129
cold sore, 64
colds, 45, 114, 169
colic, 38, 170
competitive sport, 112–113
compresses, 16–17
concentration, 35, 53–54, 96, 123
confidence, 55, 96, 167
confusion, 167
constipation, 63, 170
    pregnancy, 86
conversations, 73
cool-down spray, 113
coughs, 169
cradle cap, 38
cramps, 171
    premenstrual, 66
    sports, 114
crying, 38–39
cuts, 174
cypress, 158–159
cystitis, 63–64, 172

D

damaged hair, 138
dating, 55–56
deaf children, 47–48
deodorants, 108–109, 115
depression, 56, 79, 167
　postnatal, 91
　premenstrual, 66
dermatitis, 174
detoxifier, 127
diarrhoea, 171
digestive system, 170
dinner parties, 73
distillation, 4, 8–9
divorce, 79, 97
doctors, 30–31
douche, 17
drawer ball, 35
dry hair, 138

E

earache, 45, 169
eczema, 174
electric vaporiser, 15
emotional support, 121–123
emotions, 167–168
energising oils, 145–155
enfleurage, 9–10
epilepsy, 176
essential oils, 1–22, 141–176
eucalyptus, 146
exam nerves, 35, 54
excitement, 34
exfoliating, 133
exhaustion, 113
expression, 8
extraction, 7–10

F

facial, 19
fatal illness, 79–80
fatherhood, 97
fatigue, 77, 97, 113, 167
fear, 33, 79, 168
fennel, 146
fever, 45
first-aid kit for holidays, 94
fitness sport, 112
flatulence, 171
fleas, 36
flu, 45, 114, 169

fluid retention, 66, 174
foot massage, 49–50
footbaths, 16
frankincense, 159–160
frigidity, 80, 172
frustration, 97, 168

G

gas-liquid chromatography testing, 13
genital herpes, 64
geranium, 147–148
gifts, 34–35
glandular fever, 64
gout, 101, 171
green clay masque, 133
grief, 79, 97, 168
guilt, 168

H

haemorrhoids, 80, 174
hair
　care, 70, 110, 135–138
　loss, 136–137
　rinse, 138
　types, 138
hands, 97, 139–140
handyman, 97
hangover, 94
head, 50, 168–170
headache, 81–82, 94, 169
　premenstrual, 66
hearing-impaired child, 47–48
heart surgery, 102
heartburn, 87, 95, 171
herpes, 64, 174
high blood pressure, 101, 174, 176
holidays, 94–95
home, 74
homework, 35
honey masque, 134
housework, 74
hyperactivity, 47
hypertension, 101, 174, 176,
hysteria, 168

I

impatience, 97, 168
impotence, 103, 172
indigestion, 95, 171
inflammation, 126
influenza, 45, 114, 169

ingestion, 5–6
inhalation, 5
inhalation, steam, 22
insect bites, 95
insomnia, 34, 168

J
jealousy, 168
joints, 171–172
juniper, 148–149

K
kidneys, 176

L
labels, 11–12
labour, 89–90
lactation difficulties, 90
lamp ring, 17
laryngitis, 170
Latin names, 11
lavender, 130, 160
leg massage, 116
lemon, 149
lemongrass, 130, 150
leucorrhoea, 82
libido, 103
lice, 45
low blood pressure, 82, 174
lymphatic drainage, 18
lymphatic system, 64

M
maceration, 10
male menopause, 103
marjoram, 161
masques, 133–134, 133–135
massage, 18–20
    babies, 51
    back, 104–109
    children, 49–51
    leg, 116–121
    pregnancy, 87–88
    teenagers, 55
mastitis, 90
mature skin, 128, 132
measles, 46
meditation, 75–76
memory, 54
menopause, 82–83, 103, 172
menstruation, 172, 173
middle notes, 143

migraine, 170
mind, 167–168
moisturising, 130–132
morning sickness, 87
motherhood, 77–78
motivation, 53–54
muscles, 171–172
    tone, 114, 172
    warm-up rub, 115
mute children, 47–48
myrrh, 150

N
nails, 69–70, 139–140
nappy rash, 40
nausea, 171
negative attitude, 123
neroli, 101, 161–162
nervous system, 18
nipples, sore, 91
normal hair, 138
notes, 143–144
nurses, 30–31

O
odour, 5, 115, 142
oily hair, 138
orange, 162–163

P
pain
    labour, 89–90
    muscular, 97
    sport, 113
palpitations, 175
patchouli, 163
peppermint, 151
perfume, 20–21, 78
perspiration, 115
petitgrain, 163
pets, 36
phototoxic oils, 176
pillows, 21
pine, 152
pink clay masque, 133
PMS, 65–67, 173
positive attitude, 74
postnatal depression, 91
potpourris, 21, 57
pregnancy, 85–89, 176
premenstrual syndrome, 65–67, 173

price, 12
prostate disorders, 104
psoriasis, 67–69

R
rebellion, 56
red clay masque, 133
relationship endings, 79, 97–98
relaxation, 75–77, 155–165
reproductive system, 172–173
rheumatism, 171
romance, 74–75, 96
rose, 130, 164–165
rosemary, 152–153

S
safety, 175–176
sage, 153–154
sandalwood, 165
scalp massage, 110
scar healing, 127
school, 33, 47
sebum, 127
sensory deprived, 47–48
sexual desire, 80, 103
shampoo, 138
shaving, 55
shock, 78, 79, 136, 168
shopping for essential oils, 10–13
shoulder massage, 50
sight-impaired child, 47–48
sinusitis, 95, 170
skin, 4–5, 15, 67–69, 70–71, 108, 126–135, 173–175, 176
sleep, 94
sore losers, 123
sores, 174
sport, 111–123
sprains, 115, 172
sprays, 21, 93, 113
stamina, 115
steam inhalation, 22
steams, facial, 132
stimulating oils, 145–155
stings, 173
storage, 12
strains, 115, 172
strawberries masque 134
stretch marks, 89

study, 53–54
suicidal thoughts, 56
sunburn, 40
swab, 22
sweating, 115
synthetic oils, 10–11

T
teachers, 47
tea-tree, 100, 154
teenagers, 52–71
teething, 40, 170
throat infection, 170
thrush, 17, 84, 173
thyme, 155
time out, 75
tissue, 22
toning the skin, 129–130
tonsillitis, 46, 170
tooth fairy, 33
top notes, 143
traffic, 93
travel, 93–94
treatments, 29–30

U
urethritis, 173
urinary tract, 63, 172–173

V
vagina, 17, 82, 84, 173
vaporiser, 14–15, 35
varicose veins, 84, 175
vetiver, 165–166
visualisation exercise, 122
vomiting, 171

W
warm-up muscle rub, 115
warts, 46
wedding day, 77, 97
weight gain, 69
white clay masque, 134
whooping cough, 46–47
work, 78, 95–96

Y
yellow clay masque, 134
ylang-ylang, 166
yoghurt masque, 134